The Nurse

in Neurosurgery

The complete Guide

ALEXANDRE CAREWELL

Table of Contents

« *Neurosurgery: medical speciality devoted to surgery on the nervous system, including the brain, spinal cord and peripheral nerves.* »

Chapter 1:
INTRODUCTION TO NEUROSURGERY

Neurosurgery :
Definition and background

Neurosurgery, like a delicate dance between art and science, is the medical speciality dedicated to the study, diagnosis, surgical treatment and prevention of diseases of the nervous system. It encompasses not only the brain and spinal cord, but also the peripheral nerves that wind their way through our bodies, relaying a multitude of information every second. But how did this fascinating discipline come about?

The journey of neurosurgery through the ages takes us far into the past, long before the term itself was coined. Archaeological evidence reveals that trepanations, where part of the skull is removed, were performed over 7,000 years ago. Incredibly, these ancient procedures were sometimes followed by signs of healing, suggesting that the patient had survived the procedure. The reasons for these trepanning operations remain open to debate: were they ritual, therapeutic, or perhaps both?

Over the centuries, interest in understanding and treating the nervous system has persisted, although progress has been hampered by cultural and religious taboos, and by the limits of technology and medical knowledge. It was not until the Renaissance that anatomical studies of the brain began to gain in precision, thanks to pioneers such as Andreas Vesalius. However, neurosurgery as a distinct medical discipline only really emerged in the nineteenth century, with the advent of safer surgical techniques and a better understanding of asepsis.

15

The twentieth century saw rapid advances in neurosurgery, particularly with the introduction of medical imaging, such as computer tomography and MRI. These tools not only allowed surgeons to 'see' inside the brain before operating, but also revolutionised the diagnosis and treatment of neurological conditions.

The Journey of Neurosurgery is an ode to human curiosity and our never-ending quest for understanding. From the Stone Age to the digital age, it reflects our desire to heal and our respect for the organ that, more than any other, defines our humanity: the brain. Today, at the dawn of a new era of technological innovation and research, neurosurgery continues to push back the frontiers of what is possible, promising an even brighter future for patients around the world.

Importance of the nurse
in the neurosurgery department

The neurosurgery nurse is much more than a mere executor of medical prescriptions: he or she is the central pivot, the vigilant guardian of patients who are often in a delicate, even critical condition. Their presence, expertise and ability to intervene quickly are essential at every stage of the neurosurgical care process.

At the heart of this complex discipline, the nurse is the link between the patient, the family and the medical team. Their role extends far beyond basic clinical care. They continuously assess the patient's neurological state, interpreting subtle signs of deterioration or improvement, and adjust care accordingly. A tiny variation in consciousness or a slight difference in pupillary reactivity can be a crucial indicator for a neurosurgical patient, and it is the nurse who most often spots these changes.

In addition, the neurosurgical nurse is often faced with emergency situations, requiring rapid and precise intervention. Cerebral oedema, post-operative haemorrhage or complications due to high intracranial pressure can occur without warning, making the nurse's ability to act effectively a vital necessity.

But the importance of the nurse does not stop at direct patient care. They play an essential role in educating patients and their families, helping them to understand the disease, the surgical procedure and the recovery process. This communication is essential to establish trust, reduce anxiety and ensure effective collaboration throughout the recovery process.

The care relationship is not limited to the period of hospitalisation. Nurses also support patients in their transition to home care or other structures, ensuring that the specific needs of each patient are anticipated and met. In short, the neurosurgery nurse is a key figure, a pillar on which the success of the entire department rests. Their in-depth knowledge of the specifics of neurosurgery, combined with an ability to empathise and communicate, makes them a key player in patient care. In this surgical ballet, where every second counts and every decision can influence the final outcome, the nurse is not only an attentive observer, but also a key player in ensuring that every patient receives the best possible care.

Specific challenges and issues of the speciality

Despite its phenomenal advances, neurosurgery is not without its challenges. Like any evolving medical speciality, it is confronted with a series of obstacles and issues, from a technical, relational and ethical point of view.

Firstly, the technical aspect. The nervous system, made up of the brain, spinal cord and peripheral nerves, is mind-bogglingly complex. Surgical intervention in this delicate tangle of neurons and synapses requires millimetre precision. Tiny errors can lead to irreversible damage, making each operation both exciting and daunting. Added to this is the speed of technological change. Surgeons and their teams have to keep up to date with new methods and tools, while managing the implications of these innovations.

In terms of relationships, neurosurgery often finds itself at a crossroads between hope and reality. Managing the expectations of patients and their families, while balancing optimism with the reality of the prognosis, is a delicate exercise. The neurosurgical nurse often has to take on the role of emotional support, accompanying families through moments of joy, but also of distress.

Ethics play a vital role in this discipline. In some cases, decisions have to be made about whether or not to continue treatment, whether or not to carry out a risky operation, or how to manage end-of-life situations. The line between prolonging life and preserving quality of life is often blurred, requiring healthcare professionals to think deeply and communicate openly with patients and their families.

The economic and social stakes cannot be ignored. In many parts of the world, access to high-quality neurosurgery is limited, hampered by a lack of resources, training or infrastructure. Reducing these inequalities is a major challenge, requiring international collaboration and a strong political will.

Finally, neurosurgery, like all medical fields, is faced with the need to train the next generation of professionals. Ensuring high-quality training, while incorporating technological advances and contemporary ethical challenges, is crucial to guaranteeing the future excellence of the specialty.

Faced with these challenges, neurosurgery is constantly evolving, adapting and pushing back the boundaries. Every day, professionals in this field rise to the challenges they face with passion and dedication, guided by their unwavering commitment to their patients.

Chapter 2:
ANATOMY AND PHYSIOLOGY
OF THE NERVOUS SYSTEM

The main structures :
brain, spinal cord, nerves

The central nervous system, where the very essence of our being resides, is a complex, finely-tuned orchestra of interconnected structures. Let's take a closer look at these majestic components: the brain, the spinal cord and the nerves.

1. The brain :
At the top of this hierarchy is the brain, a spongy mass weighing around 1.4 kilograms and housing billions of neurons. It is divided into several distinct regions, each with its own responsibilities:

Cerebral cortex: The outer layer of the brain, responsible for thinking, perceiving, producing and understanding language. It is subdivided into frontal, parietal, occipital and temporal lobes.

The cerebellum: Located beneath the cortex, it plays a key role in the coordination of movement and balance.

The brain stem: Connecting the brain to the spinal cord, it manages vital functions such as breathing, heart rate and digestion.

The limbic system: Comprising the hippocampus, amygdala and hypothalamus, this is the centre of emotions, memory and associated behaviours.

2. The spinal cord :

Descending from the brain stem, it is protected by the spinal column. This nerve band transmits information between the brain and the rest of the body. It is made up of neurons and nerve tracts that transmit signals up to the brain or down to the muscles and other organs.

3. Nerves :

These bundles of nerve fibres act as the body's messengers. They carry information between the brain, the spinal cord and the rest of the body.

- *The cranial nerves:* Twelve pairs emanating directly from the brain, they control functions such as vision, hearing, smell and facial movements.
- *Spinal nerves:* Emerging from the spinal cord, they transmit information between the spinal cord and the rest of the body.
- *Peripheral nerves:* These form the network linking the rest of the body to the spinal and cranial nerves. They are responsible for sensation and movement in the limbs and other parts of the body.

These structures, with their complex interconnections, form an incredibly sophisticated network that controls almost every function in our bodies. They are both robust and delicate, capable of wonders but also vulnerable to injury and disease. This is why neurosurgery, dedicated to the preservation and restoration of these structures, is such an essential and respected discipline.

Common illnesses and diseases in neurosurgery

Neurosurgery is dedicated to the surgical management of disorders of the nervous system. The diseases and conditions encountered by neurosurgeons are many and varied, ranging from brain tumours to spinal column disorders. Let's take a look at some of the diseases and conditions most commonly treated by neurosurgeons:

1. Brain tumours :
These abnormal masses of cells can be benign or malignant. Their location, size and type determine the symptoms and treatment methods.

2. Cerebral aneurysms :
These are abnormal dilations of the walls of the blood vessels in the brain, which can lead to cerebral haemorrhage if they rupture.

3. Arteriovenous malformations (AVMs) :
These are abnormal connections between arteries and veins, mainly in the brain and spinal cord, which can cause bleeding or epileptic seizures.

4. Herniated discs :
This is the abnormal displacement of an intervertebral disc that can compress the spinal nerves, causing pain, weakness or numbness.

5. Spinal stenosis :
Narrowing of the spinal canal which can compress the spinal cord or nerves, causing neurological symptoms.

6. Craniocerebral trauma :
Brain injuries resulting from impact or trauma, ranging from mild to severe.

7. Hydrocephalus :
Abnormal accumulation of cerebrospinal fluid in or around the brain, often requiring a shunt to drain excess fluid.

8. Spinal cord tumours :
Abnormal masses developing in or around the spinal cord.

9. Cerebrovascular disease :
They include a variety of conditions, such as strokes or vessel occlusions.

10. Epilepsy :
A neurological disorder in which the brain's electrical activity becomes abnormal, causing repeated seizures.

Surgery may be considered when medication is not effective.

11. Degenerative diseases :
Such as Parkinson's disease or Huntington's disease, for which surgical interventions such as deep brain stimulation can be offered.

12. Nervous system infections :
Such as brain abscesses or empyema, which may require surgical drainage.

These conditions, although among the most common, represent only a fraction of the diseases that neurosurgeons may be called upon to treat. Each presents its own challenges and requires an individualised approach, highlighting the complexity and crucial importance of neurosurgery in patient management.

How the nervous system works: from synapse to consciousness

The nervous system is a complex network that orchestrates almost every function in our bodies, from unconscious heartbeats to the art of deep thought. To understand how we go from a simple connection between two cells to the ability to experience consciousness, it is essential to explore the structure and function of the nervous system, from the synapse to the phenomenology of consciousness itself.

1. The synapse: The first stage in neuronal communication
At the heart of the nervous system are neurons, specialised cells that transmit electrical and chemical information. When a neuron is activated, it sends an electrical signal along its axon to its endings, where it must communicate with the next neuron. This point of communication is called

the synapse. Here, chemicals called neurotransmitters are released into the synaptic cleft, where they bind to specific receptors on the neighbouring neuron, causing or inhibiting its activation.

2. Neural circuits: the synchronised dance of neurons

Billions of these synapses form immense networks of neurons. These neural circuits enable information from various sources to be integrated, processed and transmitted to other areas of the brain or body. For example, a simple touch on the skin can activate a circuit that sends information to the brain, which reacts by generating a sensation and perhaps a movement in response.

3. Brain regions: orchestrating function

The human brain is made up of many specialised regions, each playing a distinct role. The visual cortex processes visual information, while the auditory cortex processes auditory information. Other areas, such as the prefrontal cortex, are involved in abstract thinking, planning and decision-making.

4. Consciousness: The mystery of subjective experience

Consciousness is one of the great enigmas of neuroscience. How do these electrical and chemical circuits produce subjective experience, the feeling of being "oneself"? Many theories exist, from the idea that consciousness emerges from the complexity of neuronal connections, to more philosophical perspectives on the nature of existence. What we do know is that certain regions of the brain, notably the prefrontal cortex, appear to play a key role in consciousness.

5. From consciousness to cognition: The emergence of thought

Consciousness is more than just experience. It is the foundation of our cognitive capacities: reflection, memory, learning and emotion. These processes are the result of brain regions interacting in dynamic networks, constantly exchanging information and adapting according to needs and stimuli.

The journey from the signal at a synapse to the richness of human consciousness is a complex ballet of electrical, chemical and connective activities. This finely orchestrated neuronal dance is at the heart of what it means to be human, linking biology to experience, matter to spirit.

Chapter 3:
PREPARING THE PATIENT FOR SURGERY

Pre-operative assessment and full work-up

Prior to any surgical intervention, particularly in such a delicate field as neurosurgery, it is imperative to carry out a thorough pre-operative assessment. The aim of this assessment is to understand the patient's general condition, identify any potential risks associated with the operation and prepare the patient as well as possible for the surgical procedure ahead. Let's take a closer look at the stages and components of this pre-operative assessment.

1. Medical history :
The first step is to collect a full medical history from the patient, including :
- Previous illnesses
- Previous surgery
- Current medication and allergies
- Lifestyle habits (smoking, alcohol, drugs, physical activity, etc.)

2. Clinical examination :
It is crucial to assess the patient's neurological condition using a variety of tests:
- Motor and sensory tests
- Reflex evaluation
- Balance and coordination tests
- Assessment of cognitive functions

3. Additional tests :
Depending on the suspected or known pathology, various investigations are undertaken:

- **Medical imaging:** MRI (Magnetic Resonance Imaging), brain scans, angiography to visualise blood vessels, etc.
- **Electrophysiological studies:** EEG (electroencephalogram) to measure the brain's electrical activity, EMG (electromyogram) to study muscle activity, etc.
- **Blood tests:** to assess kidney and liver function, electrolyte levels and coagulation, among other things.

4. Specialist consultations :
Depending on the patient's pathology or co-morbidities, consultations with other specialists may be necessary:

- Cardiologist
- Pneumologist
- Endocrinologist
- Anaesthetist to assess anaesthetic risks

5. Psychological assessment :
Given the invasive nature of neurological surgery, it is often useful to assess the patient's mental health, their expectations of the operation and their ability to cope with pre- and post-operative stress.

6. Preoperative preparation :
Once a complete check-up has been carried out, pre-operative measurements are taken:

- Adjusting medication
- Fasting instructions
- Information on the risks and benefits of the operation
- Informed patient consent

This exhaustive pre-operative assessment ensures that each patient is treated with the utmost care, reducing the risks associated with the operation while optimising the chances of a favourable surgical outcome.

Psychological preparation
of the patient and their family

Faced with a neurosurgical operation, emotions can be particularly intense, not only for the patient himself but also for his family. Psychological preparation is therefore essential to ensure that everyone is serene and understands the situation. It can have a positive influence on the healing process, patient satisfaction and collaboration with the medical team. Here are the key steps in mentally preparing a patient and his family for a neurosurgical operation.

1. Clear and transparent information :
It is essential to provide patients and their families with detailed information on :
- The nature of the illness or injury
- The course of the operation
- Associated risks and benefits
- Anticipated post-operative effects

2. Spaces for listening and expression :
Sessions with a psychologist or psychiatrist may be offered to enable patients and their families to express their fears, doubts and hopes.

3. Support groups :
Putting patients or their families in touch with support groups or other patients who have undergone similar procedures can be beneficial. These exchanges allow them to share experiences and **advice and break down feelings of isolation.**

4. Relaxation techniques :
Methods such as meditation, deep breathing, visualisation or music can help reduce pre-operative anxiety.

5. Preparing for hospitalisation :
It is important to familiarise patients with the hospital environment and explain the various stages of their stay, from admission to discharge.

6. Family involvement :
The family plays a crucial role in providing emotional support. Reassuring them and involving them actively in the care process can reinforce the patient's sense of security.

7. Discussions on practical aspects :
Talking about logistical issues (length of hospitalisation, convalescence, possible rehabilitation, etc.) can reduce anxiety by clarifying the steps ahead.

8. Informed consent :
Ensuring that the patient fully understands the procedure and its implications, and that they give informed and voluntary consent.

9. Post-operative follow-up :
Psychological preparation does not stop at surgery. Regular follow-up with psychological support after the operation can help to manage stress, possible complications and the emotions associated with convalescence.

Careful psychological preparation is an essential element in optimising surgical results and ensuring the mental and emotional well-being of the patient and his or her family. Surgery, especially in the field of neurosurgery, is not just a technical act: it involves the whole of the human being, in his or her physical, emotional and social dimensions.

The crucial role of the nurse in the pre-operative phase

The pre-operative phase is an essential part of a patient's surgical journey, laying the foundations for a successful operation and a peaceful recovery. Nurses play a pivotal role in this phase, acting as the central link between the patient, the family and the medical team. Let's take a closer look at this multidimensional responsibility of the neurosurgical nurse during the pre-operative period.

1. Patient education and information :
The nurse is responsible for the patient's therapeutic education, ensuring that the patient understands the nature of his or her illness, the procedure, the associated risks and the foreseeable post-operative consequences. This transmission of information is adapted to each patient's level of understanding.

2. Clinical assessment :
Before the operation, the nurse carries out a clinical assessment of the patient, gathering data on his or her state of health, medical and surgical history, current treatments and any other relevant information that could influence the course of the operation.

3. Coordination with the medical team :
The nurse is often the first point of contact between the patient and the medical team. They liaise, pass on relevant information to the doctors, anaesthetists and surgeons, and ensure that all the necessary assessments are carried out.

4. Emotional preparation of the patient :
Beyond the purely clinical dimension, the nurse also listens to the patient's concerns and emotions, offering psychological support and proposing resources to help the patient manage pre-operative stress.

5. Logistics management :
The nurse organises and coordinates the various pre-operative examinations, ensures that the patient is fasting if necessary, prepares the equipment and devices required for the operation, and ensures that all pre-operative instructions are followed.

6. Prevention of complications :
Thanks to their expertise, nurses are able to identify patients at risk and implement preventive measures, such

as infection prophylaxis or the management of anticoagulant drugs.

7. Informed consent :

The nurse ensures that the patient has fully understood all the implications of the procedure and has given informed consent.

8. Family support :

The nurse is also a resource for the family, providing information, answering questions and allaying concerns.

The role of the nurse in the pre-operative phase is crucial, encompassing clinical, educational, emotional and logistical dimensions. They ensure that the patient is optimally prepared, both physically and psychologically, thereby creating the best possible conditions for a successful operation.

Chapter 4:
COMMON SURGICAL PROCEDURES IN NEUROSURGERY

Craniotomy :
techniques, indications and challenges

A craniotomy is a surgical procedure that involves opening the skull to gain access to the brain. It is commonly performed in neurosurgery to treat a variety of pathologies. In this context, let's take a look at craniotomy, its techniques, indications and associated challenges.

1. Craniotomy techniques :

Standard craniotomy: This technique involves making a skin incision on the scalp, pushing back the layers of muscle and removing a piece of bone from the skull, called a bone flap, using a special saw. Once the operation is complete, the bone flap is put back in place and fixed.

Endoscopic craniotomy: This uses an endoscope, a thin tube fitted with a camera, inserted through a small opening in the skull. This allows access to areas of the brain that are difficult to reach with a standard craniotomy.

Stereotaxis: This is a technique that uses medical images to guide surgical instruments precisely to a specific target in the brain, through a small opening.

2. Indications for craniotomy :

Brain tumours: To excise benign or malignant tumours.

Cerebral haemorrhage: To evacuate a haematoma or stop a haemorrhage.

Vascular lesions: To treat aneurysms or arteriovenous malformations.

Head injuries: To relieve intracranial pressure or repair a skull fracture.

Epilepsy: In some cases, to remove the area of the brain responsible for seizures.

Implantation of electrodes: For deep brain stimulation in conditions such as Parkinson's disease.

3. Challenges associated with craniotomy :

Note: The brain is a complex and delicate organ. Any inaccurate movement can have irreversible consequences.

Safety: It is vital to protect the brain from any potential damage, such as infection, bleeding or injury.

Length of operation: Craniotomies can be lengthy, requiring sustained concentration from the surgical team and posing anaesthetic challenges.

Communication: In certain craniotomies, the patient may be awake in order to preserve the brain's essential functions. This requires excellent communication between the surgeon, nurse, anaesthetist and patient.

Rehabilitation: The post-operative period may require intensive rehabilitation, especially if functional areas of the brain have been affected.

Craniotomy is a major operation requiring remarkable surgical expertise and team coordination. While techniques and technologies continue to evolve, craniotomy remains a mainstay of neurosurgery, offering hope to many patients with brain pathologies.

Spinal surgery :
of the intervertebral disc at fusion

Spinal surgery is a subfield of neurosurgery and orthopaedic surgery that treats diseases and injuries of the spine. These operations can range from simple discectomies to more complex procedures such as spinal fusion. Let's dive into this fascinating exploration, from the base of the intervertebral disc to fusion procedures.

1. The intervertebral disc: anatomy and function
Located between each vertebra, the intervertebral disc acts as a shock absorber, allowing spinal mobility while protecting the vertebrae from impact. It consists of a central nucleus pulposus surrounded by the annulus fibrosus, a more rigid structure.

2. Common pathologies associated with the intervertebral disc :

Herniated disc: When the nucleus pulposus protrudes through the annulus fibrosus, it can compress the nerve roots or spinal cord, causing pain and neurological dysfunction.

Disc degeneration: With age or as a result of repeated strain, the disc can wear down, losing its height and elasticity, which can cause pain and instability.

3. Common interventions on the intervertebral disc :

Discectomy: This involves removing all or part of the intervertebral disc that exerts pressure on the nerves or spinal cord. It can be performed openly or using endoscopic instruments.

Microdiscectomy: A minimally invasive form of discectomy using a microscope to visualise the surgical field.

4. Spinal fusion :

When the instability or pathology of the spine requires it, two adjacent vertebrae can be fused to form a solid unit. This process involves the use of bone grafts, plates, screws and rods to immobilise the spine while the bone consolidates.

Anterior Cervical Fusion (ACDF): This procedure approaches the spine from the front (anterior side) to remove the damaged disc and fuse the vertebrae.

Posterior fusion (PLIF or TLIF): Approached from behind, this method is commonly used for the lumbar segments of the spine.

5. Challenges and progress :

Spinal surgery, although effective, carries risks. Complications can include infection, bleeding, nerve damage or non-fusion (pseudoarthrosis). However, technological advances such as robot-assisted surgery, surgical navigation and innovative biomaterials are paving the way for safer and more effective interventions.

Spinal surgery is a complex and constantly evolving field, combining art and science to restore function, relieve pain and improve patients' quality of life. From simple intervertebral disc procedures to sophisticated fusions, each operation requires careful planning, surgical expertise and rigorous post-operative management.

Endovascular procedures : a less invasive alternative

The world of neurosurgery has been revolutionised by the advent of endovascular procedures, which offer a less invasive alternative to traditional open surgery for treating vascular pathologies of the brain. These procedures, performed inside the vessels, exploit the body's natural pathways, making it possible to treat conditions that previously required large incisions and longer recovery times. Let's take a closer look at these innovative procedures.

1. What is the endovascular procedure?
The endovascular approach is performed through the blood vessels. Using real-time imaging techniques such as fluoroscopy, the surgeon inserts catheters, guide wires and other specialised instruments through a small incision, often in the groin, and directs them to the treatment site in the brain or spinal column.

2. Advantages of endovascular procedures :
- **Less invasive:** avoids large incisions and minimises damage to surrounding tissue.
- **Faster recovery:** Patients can often leave hospital earlier and return to their normal activities more quickly.
- **Less post-operative pain:** The less invasive nature of the procedure often reduces pain and the need for medication.
- Patients not eligible for open surgery can be treated.

3. Common applications :
- **Cerebral aneurysms:** Coils can be placed inside an aneurysm to promote coagulation and prevent rupture.
- **Arteriovenous malformations (AVMs):** Injection of an embolising agent to obstruct the AVM.
- **Carotid stenosis:** use of stents to keep narrowed arteries open.
- **Mechanical thrombectomy: In the event of** a stroke, a specialised device can be used to remove a clot blocking a cerebral vessel.

4. Limitations and challenges :
- **Technical skills:** Endovascular procedures require specialised training and considerable skill.

Associated risks: Although rare, complications may include allergic reactions to the contrast medium, bleeding, infection or vascular lesions.

Accessibility: Not all pathologies are accessible or can be treated endovascularly.

5. The future of endovascular procedures :

With the development of new technologies, finer and more flexible instruments and advanced biomedical materials, the field of endovascular interventions is constantly evolving. Research continues to improve the safety, efficacy and range of treatments available.

Endovascular procedures represent a revolution in the management of neurological vascular pathologies. They offer a less invasive option, reduce morbidity and accelerate recovery, making a real difference for many patients around the world.

Chapter 5:
THE NURSE
IN THE OPERATING THEATRE

Preparing your equipment
and medical devices

In neurosurgery, the meticulous preparation of equipment and medical devices is essential to guarantee not only the effectiveness of the operation, but also the safety of the patient. From the sterile opening of packaging to the inspection of surgical instruments, each stage requires unfailing precision and in-depth knowledge of the equipment. Let's take a closer look at this essential process.

1. Needs assessment :
Before any operation, it is crucial to understand the nature of the surgery and the specific equipment requirements. This often involves close communication between the surgeon, the scrub nurse and the operating theatre staff.

2. Gathering materials :
  Checklist: An exhaustive list of the instruments, devices and supplies required is prepared and validated.
  Surgical kit: Numerous pre-assembled kits are available for specific procedures, ensuring that all essential instruments are present.
  Special equipment: Some equipment, such as surgical microscopes, navigation devices or ultrasonic aspirators, may require special preparation.

3. Sterilisation :
   Cleaning: All instruments are first thoroughly cleaned to remove debris and contaminants.
   Autoclaving: A machine called an autoclave uses pressurised steam to sterilise instruments.
   Sterility control: Biological and chemical indicators are used to guarantee sterility after autoclaving.

4. Preparation in the operating field :
   Sterile environment: The operating theatre is carefully prepared to maintain a sterile environment, including the wearing of surgical gowns, masks, caps and gloves.
   Organising instruments: The instrument nurse organises the instruments on the table logically, anticipating the surgeon's needs during the procedure.

5. Maintenance and quality control :
   Regular inspection: Instruments are regularly inspected for signs of wear, corrosion or malfunction.
   Equipment maintenance : Electronic equipment and medical devices undergo regular checks to ensure they are working properly.

6. Consumables management :
   Stock monitoring: A regular inventory of supplies is carried out to ensure the availability of essential consumables.
   Management of expired products: Products with an expiry date are monitored and disposed of in accordance with guidelines.

7. Further training :
With the rapid evolution of medical technology, it is essential that staff are trained in the latest instruments, devices and techniques. Workshops, demonstrations and formal training ensure that the team is always up to date.

The preparation of medical equipment and devices in neurosurgery is an art that demands rigour, attention to detail and ongoing training. Each instrument, each device has a precise function which, when used correctly, can make the difference between the success and failure of a procedure. The responsibility rests on the shoulders of the operating theatre team, whose dedication and expertise ensure optimal patient care.

Communication with the neurosurgeon: a perfectly orchestrated ballet

In the heart of the operating theatre, a silent dance is being performed. In this space where every millisecond counts, where precision is the watchword, communication between the nurse and the neurosurgeon is essential. It's a relationship based on mutual trust, anticipation of needs and a deep understanding of the complexity of neurosurgery. It is a ballet in which every step, every gesture, must be perfectly orchestrated to ensure the safety and success of the operation.

1. Mutual trust :
The basis of any successful collaboration between the neurosurgeon and the nurse is trust. This trust is built on years of experience, shared training and many hours spent together in the operating theatre.

2. Anticipating needs :
   Knowledge of the procedure: Nurses must have in-depth knowledge of the procedure to be carried out. This enables them to anticipate the instruments and equipment the surgeon will need at each stage.

Active listening: Even without words, the surgeon's gestures, gaze and posture give the nurse clues about immediate needs.

3. Clear, concise communication :
   Common terminology: Using standardised medical and surgical terminology helps to avoid misunderstandings.
   Constant feedback: Any request or question is immediately followed by a response, ensuring that both parties are always in sync.

4. Awareness of nuances :
   Reactivity: During surgery, unexpected situations can arise. Nurses must be able to react quickly, by providing the right tool or assisting the surgeon in the appropriate way.
   Space awareness: In the operating theatre, space is precious. Nurses must be constantly aware of their position and that of the surgeon to avoid any disruption.

5. Post-operative debriefing :
After each operation, it is beneficial for the neurosurgeon and nurse to discuss what went well and potential areas for improvement. This strengthens collaboration and ensures continuous improvement.
6. Continuing education and joint workshops :
Taking part in continuing education courses and workshops together enables the nurse and neurosurgeon to keep up to date with the latest techniques and innovations, while strengthening their collaboration.

7. Mutual respect :
Beyond verbal and non-verbal communication, mutual respect is fundamental. Each member of the team has a

crucial role to play, and recognition of each other's contribution is essential to successful collaboration.

Communication between the nurse and the neurosurgeon is a delicate art, a meticulously orchestrated choreography which, when well executed, becomes a harmonious dance, where every movement is fluid, every request is anticipated and every action is perfectly synchronised. It is this level of collaboration and mutual understanding that guarantees the best results for the patient and the success of each operation.

Ensuring the patient's safety and well-being during the operation

In neurosurgery, the margin for error is minimal. Each operation is a complex challenge requiring technical expertise, but also a constant concern for the patient's safety and well-being. This responsibility falls not only to the neurosurgeon, but also to the entire medical team, particularly the nurse. Let's take a closer look at this crucial role, a veritable protective shield for the patient, right at the heart of the action.

1. Preparation: an essential stage
    Identity check: Before starting, it is essential to confirm the patient's identity, the planned procedure and the surgical site.
    Monitoring equipment: The nurse ensures that all monitoring devices (ECG, pulse oximetry, blood pressure monitor) are in place and working properly.
2. Constant surveillance :
    Monitoring vital signs: The nurse constantly monitors the patient's vital signs, detecting any irregularities or signs of instability.

Anomaly alert: Any change in vital signs, oxygenation or neurological response is immediately reported to the surgeon and anaesthetist.

3. Pain management :

Administration of analgesics: Depending on the anaesthetist's instructions, the nurse may administer analgesics to ensure the patient's comfort.

Monitoring for side effects: The patient's reaction to the medication is closely monitored to prevent any adverse effects.

4. Prevention of complications :

Patient positioning: The nurse ensures that the patient is optimally positioned to avoid skin lesions, nerve compressions or other complications.

Infection prevention : The use of a sterile drape, compliance with asepsis protocols and monitoring of the incision are key steps in minimising the risk of infection.

5. Communication with the team :

Passing on information: The nurse plays a central role in communication between the surgeon, anaesthetist and other members of the medical team.

Emotional support: In some cases, the nurse can also provide emotional support for the patient, especially if the patient is conscious during part of the procedure.

6. Preparing for the post-operative phase :

Equipment ready: Before the end of the operation, the nurse prepares all the equipment needed for the patient's immediate recovery, including respiratory assistance devices and medication.

The nurse is the patient's silent guardian angel throughout the neurosurgical procedure. He or she ensures that every aspect of the patient's safety and well-being is taken into account, ensuring that the surgical experience is as safe and comfortable as possible. This task requires a combination of technical skill, attention to detail, and genuine empathy for each patient.

Chapter 6:
POST-OPERATIVE CARE

Monitoring vital signs and potential complications

Monitoring vital signs during neurosurgery is not a passive task. It is an active and constant quest to anticipate and prevent any problems that could endanger the patient's life. For the nurse, this means not only monitoring screens, but also having a deep understanding of the patient, their condition, and the potential complications that may arise.

1. Understanding vital signs :
    - **Heart rate:** A significant increase or decrease may indicate stress, haemorrhage or a side effect of medication.
    - **Blood pressure:** Low blood pressure may suggest haemorrhage, while high blood pressure may be a response to stress or pain.
    - **Breathing:** Changes in breathing rate may signal respiratory distress or obstruction.
    - **Temperature:** Hypothermia or hyperthermia can affect cerebral metabolism and blood flow.
    - **Oxygen saturation:** A drop in oxygen saturation can indicate hypoxia, compromising the brain and other vital organs.
2. Recognition of neurological complications :
    - **Changes in level of consciousness:** Sudden drowsiness, agitation or convulsions may signal brain damage or another complication.
    - **Pupillary responses:** Dilated or unresponsive pupils may indicate increased intracranial pressure or brain damage.

Abnormal movements: Tremors, spasms or paralysis may suggest nerve damage or other complications.

3. Prevent cardiovascular complications :

Embolism: Careful monitoring for signs of embolism, such as chest pain or dyspnoea, is crucial.

Cardiac arrest: Rapid recognition and intervention in the event of cardiac arrest can mean the difference between life and death.

4. Monitoring wound condition :

Haemorrhage: Excessive bleeding may indicate internal haemorrhage or a coagulation problem.

Signs of infection: Redness, swelling or discharge of abnormal fluid should be reported immediately.

5. Post-operative complications :

Cerebral oedema: Swelling of the brain can compress vital structures and increase intracranial pressure.

Cerebrospinal fluid fistulas: Leakage of clear fluid from the wound may indicate a fistula.

6. Communication with the team :

Reporting abnormalities: Any change in vital signs or any other suspicious sign should be reported immediately to the medical team.

Accurate documentation: Keeping detailed records makes it possible to monitor patient progress and anticipate complications.

Monitoring vital signs and potential complications in neurosurgery is a demanding task that requires vigilance, expertise and responsiveness. Nurses must be equipped not only with medical knowledge, but also with keen intuition, always on the lookout for the slightest signs of distress or complications. This role is essential to guarantee the best possible outcome for each patient.

Pain management :
from pharmacology to practice

Pain, often described as a subjective and unpleasant experience, is a major concern in neurosurgery. Managing it properly not only promotes faster recovery, but also improves patients' quality of life. For the neurosurgical nurse, understanding pain mechanisms, pharmacological options and optimal care practices is essential.

1. Understanding pain :
   Pain mechanisms: Understanding the differences between nociceptive, neuropathic and inflammatory pain.
   Pain assessment: Use of pain scales, behavioural observations and patient feedback for accurate assessment.
2. Pharmacological options :
   Non-opioid analgesics: Paracetamol, NSAIDs (non-steroidal anti-inflammatory drugs) and their role in relieving moderate pain.
   Opioids: Morphine, oxycodone, fentanyl and others: understanding their mechanisms of action, indications and potential side effects.
   Adjuvants : Medications such as tricyclic antidepressants, antiepileptics and muscle relaxants, used to treat neuropathic pain or increase the effectiveness of analgesics.
3. Administration techniques :
   Routes of administration: Oral, intravenous, epidural, intramuscular and others.
   Patient-controlled analgesia (PCA) pumps: How they work, indications, benefits and challenges.
4. Non-pharmacological practices :
   Physical therapies: such as heat, cold, massage and transcutaneous electrical stimulation (TENS).

Psychological interventions: relaxation techniques, meditation, cognitive-behavioural therapies.

Complementary approaches: Acupuncture, aromatherapy, music therapy.

5. Monitoring and evaluation :

Side effects: Recognising and managing the common side effects of analgesic drugs.

Regular reassessment: Ensure that pain is periodically assessed so that management can be adapted accordingly.

Preventing dependence: Recognising the signs of potential dependence, especially with the use of opioids, and preventive measures.

6. Communication and education :

Patient education: informing patients about medicines, their effects and how to manage pain effectively at home.

Communication with the medical team: sharing information about the patient's pain level, the medicines administered and their observed effects.

7. Ethics and pain management :

Informed consent: Ensuring that the patient understands the benefits and risks associated with treatment.

Patient rights: Recognition of the patient's fundamental right to adequate pain relief.

Pain management in neurosurgery is a combination of art and science. It requires a deep understanding of the mechanisms of pain, a thorough knowledge of the pharmacological options available, and a holistic, individualised approach to each patient. The nurse plays a central role in this management, acting as a link between the patient, the pain and the medical team.

The essential role of the nurse in patient rehabilitation and support

Post-surgery is a crucial period, marked not only by physical recovery, but also by psychological recovery. Rehabilitation is the process by which patients regain their independence and quality of life. The nurse, in addition to his or her clinical skills, becomes an essential pillar in the patient's reconstruction, guiding him or her through each stage of recovery.

1. Post-operative assessment :
   Clinical status: Monitoring vital signs and the surgical wound, and early detection of complications.
   Pain assessment: Ensuring optimum comfort while avoiding excessive medication.

2. Early mobilisation :
   Encouraging activity: Helping the patient to resume basic movements, which are essential to avoid complications such as thrombosis or post-operative pneumonia.
   Physical therapy: In collaboration with physiotherapists, facilitate adapted exercises to strengthen muscles and improve coordination.

3. Psychological support :
   Active listening: Allowing patients to express their fears, anxieties and hopes.
   Information: Explain to patients how their rehabilitation is progressing, the progress they expect to make and the next steps to be taken.
   Stress management: relaxation techniques, meditation or group therapy.

4. Education and autonomy :
Training in everyday procedures: Teaching patients how to manage their wounds, their medication and any other necessary care.

Promoting self-management: Encouraging patients to take charge of their health and recognise signs of improvement or complications.

5. Social and family reintegration :

Family counselling: Helping the family to understand the healing process and the patient's needs.

Referral to support groups: Encouraging exchanges with other patients who have been through similar experiences.

Planning the return home: Ensuring that the patient's environment is adapted to their needs and level of autonomy.

6. Medical follow-up planning :

Post-operative appointments: Organise regular consultations with the neurosurgeon or other specialists.

Coordination with other health professionals: Working closely with physiotherapists, occupational therapists and social workers.

7. Health promotion and prevention :

Lifestyle advice: Encourage a healthy diet, regular physical activity and smoking cessation.

Education on warning signs: Inform patients of the symptoms to watch out for and the importance of regular medical check-ups.

Nurses play a multifaceted role in post-neurosurgical rehabilitation. They are not only the guarantor of clinical care, but also a companion, an educator and a valuable ally for the patient and his or her family. In this journey from convalescence to full recovery, the nurse is often the compass that guides the patient, reassuring and supporting them every step of the way.

Chapter 7:
EMOTIONAL CHALLENGES
AND PSYCHOLOGICAL

Managing hopes and patients' fears

Navigating the stormy waters of neurosurgery is not only a physical challenge, but also an emotional one for patients. They often find themselves in a whirlwind of emotions, torn between the hope of a better life after the operation and the fear of complications or even an unknown outcome. In this context, the nurse acts as a lighthouse, lighting the way and calming the inner storms.

To understand patients' hopes is to touch their very essence, their dreams of a pain-free life, regained mobility or simply better days. These hopes are sometimes the fuel that drives them forward, to accept a risky procedure or endure arduous therapies. However, these hopes can sometimes be exaggerated, based on unrealistic expectations or anecdotal evidence. The nurse must then guide this hope, modulate it without shattering it. It's a delicate dance between compassion, objective information and support.

At the same time, the fears are just as real, lurking in the shadows. Fear of the unknown, of change, or even of losing a part of oneself. These apprehensions, although natural, can hinder healing, create stress or even lead a patient to abandon a potentially life-saving treatment. At such times, the nurse takes on the role of protector, allaying these fears by listening, educating and reassuring. The aim is not to minimise these fears, but to confront them together, armed with knowledge and understanding.

It is in this complex mix of hope and fear that nurses weave a unique relationship with each patient. A relationship based on trust, transparency and caring. Every day, they are the silent witnesses of whispered dreams and confided worries. And every day, they strive to build a bridge between these two worlds, bringing hope closer to reality while keeping the shadows of fear at bay.

Managing patients' hopes and fears is not just a simple task, it's an art, it's a responsibility, it's an honour. And through this unwavering dedication, the nurse often becomes the guardian of souls, the bearer of light in the darkest moments of neurosurgery.

Supporting families in difficult times

When illness strikes, it doesn't just affect the patient; it also sends shockwaves through the whole family. Relatives, often distraught and overwhelmed by emotion, find themselves confronted with a reality they had never imagined. In these dark hours, the nurse takes on a role that goes well beyond that of carer: he or she becomes a support, a guide and sometimes even a refuge for these torn families.

The hospital, with its sterile corridors and dim lights, can be an intimidating place. Every beep of a monitor, every whispered discussion between health professionals can cause growing anxiety in loved ones. This is where the nurse comes in, offering not only clear and transparent information, but also an attentive ear, ready to listen, reassure and console.

Every family is unique, with its own set of values, beliefs and needs. Some are looking for precise medical details, others simply need a space to cry, and still others are looking for hope, even the smallest hope. To discern these needs is to plunge into the heart of the human condition, to perceive vulnerability and respond with compassion.

Support is not limited to the time spent in hospital. The nurse also accompanies the family on their return home, when the patient and their loved ones have to adapt to a new normality. They help them navigate the maze of post-operative care, address their night-time concerns and direct them to resources and support groups.

Difficult times are also moments of great intimacy. Moments when, sitting at the bedside of a sleeping patient, a parent confides his or her deepest fears, when a spouse expresses gratitude between sobs, when a child, eyes full of tears, asks questions to which even adults have no answers. In these fragile moments, nurses offer more than clinical skills; they offer their humanity.

Supporting families through difficult times means recognising that healing is not just about the body, but also encompasses the mind, the soul and the heart. It's a delicate dance between science and empathy, where the nurse, hand in hand with the family, charts a path of hope through the darkness.

The resilience of the nurse : preventing burnout

The hospital environment, with its frenetic pace and constant demands, is a world apart. In the midst of this melee, nurses move forward, juggling patients' needs, medical demands and the often intense emotions that run through the hospital corridors. Faced with these daily challenges, nurses' resilience is put to the test, and the threat of burnout looms on the horizon.

Burnout is insidious. It often begins with simple signs: fatigue that doesn't go away, growing irritability, a feeling of detachment. But if these signs are ignored, they can worsen, leading to disillusionment, diminished professional capacity and, ultimately, emotional and physical collapse.

So how can nurses cultivate their resilience in the face of these ever-present challenges? Firstly, by recognising the importance of self-care. Yes, nurses are a pillar for their patients and colleagues, but it's just as crucial that they take time to recharge their batteries. This can take the form of regular breaks, moments of meditation or relaxation, hobbies or activities that they enjoy outside work.

Communication is also essential. Talking about your feelings and sharing your experiences with colleagues or loved ones can offer perspective and relief. What's more, it's vital to recognise one's limitations and to ask for help when necessary. No one is an island, and mutual support within the medical team is often the key to overcoming the most difficult periods.

Finally, ongoing training and updating of skills can provide a sense of mastery and achievement, boosting nurses' self-confidence.

Resilience, like burnout, is not a fixed state, but rather a continuum. At each stage, nurses have a choice: to allow themselves to be overwhelmed by the waves of demands and emotions, or to learn to surf them, to master them, thereby strengthening their resistance to future storms.

In the face of burnout, nurses' resilience is not a luxury, it's a necessity. It's the shield that protects against the onslaughts of everyday life, enabling nurses to continue to provide the quality care their patients need, while preserving their own well-being.

Chapter 8:
TEAMWORK IN NEUROSURGERY

Interaction with other medical and surgical specialities

The world of neurosurgery, with its inherent complexity, cannot exist in isolation. It evolves within a dynamic network of medical and surgical specialities, forming a mesh of expertise that, when combined, guarantees patients comprehensive and optimal care. In this multidisciplinary ballet, the nurse plays an essential role as a link, ensuring that the interaction between the various players is fluid and coherent.

Take, for example, a patient suffering from a brain tumour. In addition to the neurosurgical team, a number of other specialities may be involved: oncologists to assess and treat the cancerous aspect of the tumour, radiologists for diagnostic images, neurologists to assess neurological function, and physiotherapists for post-operative rehabilitation. In this conglomeration of expertise, the nurse acts as a point of reference for the patient, facilitating communication between these different services.

Interactions are not just limited to the medical aspect. Nurses also play a crucial role in coordinating with other hospital services, such as pharmacy, nutrition and psychology. Understanding the specific needs of each patient, and knowing which expert to refer to and when, is an art that nurses master brilliantly.

In addition, the relationship with other specialties is not only reactive, but also proactive. Neurosurgical nurses regularly attend multidisciplinary meetings, seminars and workshops. These exchanges enable them to keep abreast of the latest advances in other fields, expand their knowledge and establish solid professional relationships.

The nurse's ability to interact effectively with other specialties not only benefits the patient. It also enhances the reputation and quality of care offered by the neurosurgery department. Every successful interaction, every bridge built between disciplines, is another step towards medical excellence.

So, over and above technical skills and compassion, the art of interaction is one of the keys to success for the neurosurgical nurse. In this complex medical chessboard, they become the architects of integrated care, ensuring that each piece finds its place, and that the patient always remains at the heart of the system.

Effective communication with anaesthetists, radiologists and other healthcare professionals

Neurosurgery, by its very nature, is a discipline that requires millimetre precision, flawless synchronisation and unparalleled interdisciplinary coordination. It is a field where the margin for error is reduced to a minimum. At the centre of this medical dance is the nurse, often playing the role of conductor, ensuring that each health professional plays his or her part in harmony. Effective communication between the nurse and other healthcare professionals, particularly anaesthetists and radiologists, is therefore essential.

The anaesthetist, for example, is a crucial ally during a neurosurgical operation. Long before the first scalpel touches the skin, the nurse works closely with the anaesthetist to prepare the patient. This involves understanding the patient's specific anaesthetic needs, anticipating any risks and discussing the particularities of the forthcoming operation. The nurse's close relationship with the patient provides essential information about the patient's emotional state, history and expectations, enabling the anaesthetist to personalise his or her approach.

Radiologists, for their part, are the eyes that allow us to glimpse the invisible. The images they provide are often the guide that directs the surgeon through the labyrinth of the nervous system. The nurse facilitates this collaboration by ensuring that the patient is well prepared for the various imaging procedures, relaying the surgeon's concerns to the radiologist, and ensuring that the images produced meet the specific needs of the operation.

But communication is not just about verbal exchanges. It also involves understanding the language of other disciplines, and correctly interpreting signs, gestures and expressions. Nurses need to be active listeners, sensitive to what is not always said out loud, but which is just as important.

Other healthcare professionals, such as physiotherapists, nutritionists, psychologists and social workers, are all partners with whom nurses must interact on a daily basis. The success of this collaboration depends on mutual respect, trust and, above all, recognition of the value of each profession.

At the end of the day, communication isn't just about a skill; it's an art. And in the world of neurosurgery, where every moment counts, every detail matters, the nurse excels as a communication artist, building bridges between disciplines, harmonising care, and ensuring that the patient receives the best possible, coordinated and holistic treatment.

The role of technicians, Caregivers and other members support staff

Within the medical ecosystem, neurosurgery, although an extremely precise field, cannot operate in a vacuum. The efficiency and success of a neurosurgery department depend on synergy, a delicate balance between different professionals. While surgeons, anaesthetists and nurses are often seen as the main players, the role of technicians, Caregivers and other support staff is just as crucial. They are the silent but indispensable pillars of this structure.

Technicians, for example, are often the experts in cutting-edge surgical equipment. Whether it's calibrating an operating microscope, preparing navigation equipment or adjusting an imaging device, their expertise is invaluable. They ensure that every tool and every machine is working at optimum efficiency, enabling surgeons to operate with unrivalled precision. Their role often extends beyond simple maintenance; they are also trainers, informers, and sometimes even innovators, suggesting improvements or adaptations.

As for the Caregivers, they are the guardians of patients' well-being. In the hustle and bustle of an operating theatre or care unit, they are often the first to notice a change, a variation, a worry. Their role goes far beyond simple assistance: they provide hygiene care, help with mobilisation, offer emotional support and often act as an intermediary between the patient, their family and the medical team. Their proximity and sensitivity make them essential observers and front-line workers.

Other support staff, whether administrative, logistical or cleaning, also play a key role. They ensure that every cog in the system works in harmony. The secretary who organises appointments, the logistician who makes sure that operating theatres are available, the cleaner who ensures that rooms are sterile, all contribute to the success of operations.

In this medical ballet, each professional, whatever their function, is a key player. The nurse, aware of this interdependence, works closely with each of them, valuing their work, building bridges of communication and guaranteeing the cohesion of the team. Because in neurosurgery, every detail counts, every second is precious, and it's thanks to the sum of everyone's skills and dedication that excellence is achieved.

Chapter 9:
TOOLS AND TECHNOLOGIES IN NEUROSURGERY

Presentation of the cutting-edge equipment used in the operating theatre

Neurosurgery, a discipline at the frontiers of what is possible, has always been a field in which technology and innovation play a central role. The complex challenges of this speciality require cutting-edge equipment to ensure the precision, safety and efficiency of operations. At the heart of this quest is the operating theatre, a veritable technological sanctuary, where every instrument plays a key role in the success of procedures.

The **operating microscope is one of** the emblematic tools of neurosurgery. With its exceptional magnification capacity and often coupled with fluorescence technologies, it enables surgeons to distinguish delicate nerve structures, blood vessels and pathological tissues with unequalled clarity.

Surgical navigation systems, comparable to a GPS for the surgeon, offer real-time visualisation of the position of instruments in relation to the patient's anatomy. Coupled with advanced imaging software, these systems enable a less invasive approach, reducing risks and speeding up recovery.

Intraoperative neuromonitoring is another revolutionary innovation. It enables live monitoring of the electrical activity of the brain, nerves or spinal cord during the operation. This gives the surgeon instant feedback on neurological function, minimising the risk of damage.

Robot-assisted surgery is also beginning to gain ground. These robots, directed by surgeons, combine mechanical precision with human flexibility, enabling even more precise operations and minimising surgeon fatigue.

Neurosurgical endoscopy is another key piece of equipment. Using fine cameras and instruments, it allows access to areas of the brain or spinal column that were previously difficult to reach, all through small incisions.

Finally, **ultrasonic coagulation equipment** and **surgical lasers** have revolutionised the way tissue is cut and coagulated, reducing bleeding and improving visibility during the operation.

This equipment, although incredibly sophisticated, is only a tool. Their true potential is realised in the hands of surgeons and trained medical teams, and it is often the nurses who ensure that they are properly prepared, maintained and used to optimum effect. It is in this alchemy between people and technology that the magic of modern neurosurgery comes to life, constantly pushing back the boundaries of what is possible.

Advances in medical imaging and their importance

Medical imaging has been the mainstay of many medical disciplines since its inception. It has undergone dazzling technological advances in recent decades, constantly redefining the limits of our understanding and our ability to diagnose, plan and treat. In neurosurgery, these advances are particularly crucial, as they offer a precise and detailed window onto one of the most complex systems in the human body: the nervous system.

Magnetic Resonance Imaging (MRI) has been one of the most revolutionary advances. Offering detailed images of the brain, spinal cord and peripheral nerves without the need for radiation, it has become indispensable for spotting tumours, vascular anomalies or areas of inflammation. Functional MRI, a variant, can even map brain activity in real time, identifying the regions involved in language, movement or sensation.

Positron Emission Tomography (PET), although less commonly used in neurosurgery, provides metabolic information about tissues. It is particularly useful for differentiating between healthy and diseased tissue, as in the case of tumours.

Computed tomography (CT scan), using X-rays, provides cross-sectional images of the body and is often used to detect bleeding, fractures or masses.

Vessel-specific **angiography** is crucial in neurosurgery for visualising the vascular network of the brain and spinal cord. Advances such as CT or MRI angiography have made it possible to obtain these images without introducing a catheter into the vascular system.

Magnetic Resonance Elastography is a more recent technique that measures the rigidity or elasticity of tissues, offering potentially valuable information on conditions such as tumours or scarring.

Beyond these technologies, what is truly revolutionary is the way in which they can be combined and used simultaneously. For example, the fusion of MRI and CT images enables complete visualisation of anatomical structures and pathological features.

The importance of these advances in imaging for neurosurgery is colossal. Not only do they guide diagnosis, but they also play an essential role in surgical planning, helping surgeons to define safe trajectories and avoid vital structures. During the operation, intraoperative imaging gives the surgeon real-time feedback, increasing the precision and safety of the operation.

These advances have also strengthened the role of nurses. Understanding imaging techniques, preparing patients for examinations, monitoring them during procedures and interpreting results for post-operative follow-up are all aspects that require specialist nursing expertise. So, at every stage, from discovery to application, medical imaging and neurosurgery are advancing hand in hand, continually transforming the outlook and potential of the medical field.

How nurses can keep up with technological developments

Technological developments in medicine, and neurosurgery in particular, are rapid and constant. It promises better interventions, faster recovery and more personalised care for patients. But for healthcare professionals, this constant evolution also means a constant need for training and adaptation. For nurses, whose role is central to patient care, keeping up to date is essential to ensuring optimal care. Here's how to do it:

Continuing education: Most medical institutions offer continuing education programmes for their employees. Regular participation in these courses enables nurses to familiarise themselves with the latest equipment, techniques and protocols.

Workshops and seminars: Many professional organisations organise workshops and seminars dedicated to the latest technological advances. These events are also excellent opportunities to network with experts and peers.

Specialist certifications: Obtaining certification in a specific area of neurosurgery or medical imaging can help nurses deepen their skills and keep abreast of the latest techniques.

Attending conferences: Medical conferences, whether national or international, provide a wealth of information on the latest research, innovations and technologies.

Regular reading: Specialist magazines, medical journals and online publications are excellent resources for keeping up to date. Subscribing to relevant journals or specialist newsletters can help filter information.

Hospital working groups and committees: Participating in groups or committees dedicated to the evaluation and adoption of new technologies gives you a direct insight into innovations and enables you to play an active part in their implementation.

Interdisciplinary collaboration: Regular exchanges with colleagues from other specialities, such as radiologists, neurosurgeons or biomedical technicians, enrich our understanding of new technologies and their application.

E-learning and online courses: With the boom in online training, many specialised courses can now be accessed remotely, offering flexibility and accessibility.

Professional social networks: Platforms such as LinkedIn or specialist forums can be excellent ways of following opinion leaders, sharing resources and exchanging best practice.

Adaptability and open-mindedness: More than a technical skill, the ability to adapt and embrace change is crucial. Openness to new things and curiosity are major assets.

Faced with this technological effervescence, nurses are not just passive recipients. Through their commitment, ongoing training and passion for patient care, they play an active role in the adoption and optimisation of these innovations, ensuring the best possible care for their patients.

Chapter 10:
EMERGENCY MANAGEMENT IN NEUROSURGERY

Intra-operative complications and how to manage them

During neurosurgical operations, there is always a risk of complications. These complications can vary in severity, and their management requires preparation, rapid action and close collaboration between all members of the surgical team. Here is an exploration of common complications and strategies for managing them.

Haemorrhage :

Identification: Rapid blood loss, a fall in blood pressure or an increase in pulse may indicate haemorrhage.

Management: Haemorrhage must be controlled immediately by identifying the source and using haemostatic agents, sutures or clips. The anaesthetist must compensate for blood loss with transfusions if necessary.

Injury to a major blood vessel :

Identification: Direct observation, abnormal pulsations or sudden onset of bleeding.

Management: Immediate repair is necessary, either by suturing the vessel or using vascular clips.

Damage to nerves or neural structures:

Identification: Direct observation or abnormal response during intra-operative nerve stimulation.

Management: Avoid any additional tension or pressure on the area. If a lesion is identified, consult the neurosurgeon to assess the best restorative approach.

Reaction to anaesthesia :

Identification: changes in vital signs, respiratory arrest, allergies.

Management: The anaesthetist must quickly identify and treat the problem, whether by modifying the medication, administering opposing agents or taking other measures.

Infection :

Identification: Signs of inflammation, high temperature, purulence.

Management: administer antibiotics, maintain a strict sterile field and, if possible, identify and eliminate the source of infection.

Equipment problems :

Identification: Malfunction or breakdown of devices or instruments.

Management: Always have back-up equipment available. Regularly train staff in fault detection and management.

Increase in intracranial   pressure :

Identification: Changes in vital signs, abnormal responses to stimulation, visible brain swelling.

Management: Administer medication to reduce pressure, such as osmotic diuretics. Consider decompression if necessary.

Respiratory complications :

Identification: Insufficient oxygenation, increased CO2, breathing difficulties.

Management: Ensure adequate ventilation, reassess intubation or ventilation, administer bronchodilator medication if necessary.

Each complication has its own subtleties, and the response must be tailored to the specific situation. Preparation before surgery, including simulation of emergency scenarios, ongoing training and transparent communication between team members, are essential to managing these complications effectively. In a delicate environment such as neurosurgery, every second counts, and rapid, coordinated intervention can make the difference between a positive outcome and a tragic event.

Post-operation emergencies: haematomas, infections, etc.

The post-operative period is critical in the care of a patient who has undergone neurosurgery. A number of complications can arise, and the ability of the care team to identify them quickly and act accordingly is essential. Here is an overview of common post-operative emergencies and strategies for managing them:

Post-operative haematomas :
Identification: Sudden increase in pain, swelling at the surgical site, changes in neurological signs, deterioration in vital signs.
Management: If a haematoma is suspected, immediate imaging is required. Evacuation surgery may be required depending on the size and location.
Infections :
Identification: Redness, warmth, swelling or purulent discharge at the surgical site, fever, chills or changes in neurological status.
Management: Cultures of any suspicious discharge, administration of broad-spectrum antibiotics while awaiting results, and

sometimes re-operation to clean the infected area.

Cerebrospinal fluid (CSF) fistulas :

Identification: Clear discharge from the wound, signs of meningitis, or symptoms of reduced CSF pressure such as postural headaches.

Management: Bed rest, possibly external compression, and in some cases re-operation to close the leak.

Respiratory complications :

Identification: Difficulty breathing, cyanosis, oxygen desaturation.

Management: oxygen therapy, positioning to facilitate breathing, aspiration of secretions if necessary, and assessment by a pneumologist or anaesthetist.

Deep vein thrombosis (DVT) and pulmonary embolism :

Identification: Swelling, pain or redness of a limb, shortness of breath, chest pain.

Management: Diagnostic evaluation with venous ultrasound or pulmonary scintigraphy, anticoagulation for treatment.

Neurological deficits :

Identification: Weakness, paralysis, numbness, difficulty speaking or understanding, blurred vision.

Management: Immediate neurological assessment, brain imaging to identify the cause, appropriate medical or surgical interventions.

Drug reactions :

Identification: Skin rash, breathing difficulties, cardiac abnormalities, confusion.

Management: Stop the suspect drug, treat specific symptoms, monitor vital signs closely.

Dehydration and electrolyte imbalances :

Identification: Confusion, dry mouth, weakness, abnormal heart rhythms.

Management: Rehydration, correction of imbalances, regular monitoring of electrolyte levels.

Vigilance is the watchword in the post-operative period. Constant monitoring, regular assessment of the patient's condition and open communication between all members of the medical team are crucial to anticipating and effectively managing any complications that may arise.

Rapid response protocols and decision-making in critical situations

Neurosurgery is a field where emergency situations can rapidly evolve into life-threatening crises. Rapid and effective response is essential. This requires a well-trained team, familiar with rapid intervention protocols and capable of making informed decisions in real time.

Initial assessment :

As soon as an alarm sign appears, an immediate assessment of vital signs and neurological status is imperative.

Communication is key: it is essential to inform the neurosurgeon, anaesthetist and all the medical team involved as soon as possible.

Protocol for intracranial hypertension (ICHT) :

Signs: Severe headache, nausea, vomiting, disturbed consciousness, dilated pupils.

Actions: Elevate the head of the bed, administer osmotic drugs such as mannitol, consider assisted ventilation to reduce PCO2, and carry out brain imaging.

Seizure protocol :

Signs: Abnormal movements, loss of consciousness.

Actions: Ensure a clear airway, administer anticonvulsants such as diazepam or lorazepam, set up continuous EEG monitoring if available.

Shock protocol :

Signs: Hypotension, tachycardia, cold clammy skin.

Actions: Administer intravenous fluids, assess the cause of shock (haemorrhage, infection, anaphylactic reaction) and treat accordingly.

Protocol for apnea or respiratory distress :

Signs: Absence of breathing, cyanosis, agitation.

Actions: Clear the airway, administer oxygen, consider intubation and mechanical ventilation.

Post-operative emergency protocol :

Signs: Active bleeding, neurological deterioration, sudden swelling.

Actions: Immediate assessment by the surgeon, preparation for a possible re-operation, imaging to determine the cause.

Heart failure   protocol :

Signs: Shortness of breath, pulmonary oedema, irregular heartbeat.

Actions: Semi-sitting position, administer medication such as diuretics, consider cardiac assessment.

Emergency protocol in the event of an anaesthetic accident :

Signs: Hypoxia, cardiac arrest, allergic reaction.

Actions: Stop administration of any suspect drugs, start CPR, administer resuscitation drugs.

Having rapid response protocols in place provides the medical team with a clear roadmap in potentially chaotic situations. However, beyond the protocols, the team's ability to collaborate effectively, communicate clearly and trust each other's expertise is just as crucial. Regular simulations and training can help to reinforce these skills and prepare the team to manage crises with skill and confidence.

Chapter 11:
MINIMUM INTERVENTIONS
IN NEUROSURGERY

Stereotaxis: principles and applications

Stereotaxy is a surgical technique that enables a region of the brain to be precisely targeted using a system of three-dimensional coordinates. Born of collaboration between neurosurgery and neurology, it is at the forefront of minimally invasive procedures. Stereotactic procedures are commonly used in the treatment of various neurological disorders, and the precision they offer is essential for preserving vital brain structures.

1. Fundamental principles of stereotaxy :
   - **Coordinate system** : Stereotaxy is based on the creation of a fixed coordinate system, often using a metal frame attached to the patient's head. This frame serves as a reference point for locating target areas within the brain.
   - **Imaging**: Imaging techniques such as MRI (magnetic resonance imaging) or CT (computed tomography) are used to obtain detailed images of the brain. These images are then merged with the coordinate system to plan the operation.
   - **Precision**: The precise nature of stereotaxy allows neurosurgeons to reach target areas with a minimum margin of error, which is crucial for preventing damage to adjacent structures.

2. Common applications :
   - **Surgery for movement disorders**: Stereotaxy is often used in the treatment of Parkinson's disease,

dystonia and essential tremor. It may involve implanting electrodes for deep brain stimulation (DBS) or performing a thalamotomy or pallidotomy.

Brain biopsy: When suspicious lesions are detected in the brain, a stereotactic biopsy can be performed to take a tissue sample for analysis, while minimising the risks.

Epilepsy surgery: Stereotaxy can be used to target and treat the areas of the brain responsible for epileptic seizures.

Treatment of tumours: Stereotaxy can be used to administer targeted radiotherapy, known as radiosurgery, to brain tumours. Gamma Knife and CyberKnife are examples of devices that use this technology.

Draining abscesses or cysts : Using stereotaxy, surgeons can precisely drain abscesses or cysts in the brain.

3. Benefits and challenges :

Minimally invasive: One of the main virtues of stereotaxy is that it allows access to the brain without the need for large incisions or extensive craniotomies.

Risk reduction: By precisely targeting the area of interest, stereotaxy minimises the risk of damage to vital brain structures.

Challenges: Despite its precision, stereotaxy requires considerable expertise and meticulous planning. Correct interpretation of the images is essential, and any movement by the patient can compromise accuracy.

Stereotaxy has revolutionised neurosurgery, offering innovative ways of treating neurological conditions with unrivalled precision. As with all surgical procedures, communication between the nurse, neurosurgeon and the rest of the medical team is essential to ensure the best outcome for the patient.

Neuroendoscopy : techniques and benefits

Neuroendoscopy is a medical procedure that uses an endoscope to visualise and intervene on the internal structures of the brain and spinal column. It represents a significant advance in the field of neurosurgery, offering a less invasive approach to treating a variety of conditions. As with any cutting-edge medical technology, neuroendoscopy requires a thorough understanding of its techniques and benefits if it is to be applied successfully.

1. Neuroendoscopy techniques :

Rigid and flexible endoscopes: Endoscopes can be rigid or flexible. Rigid endoscopes are often used for the cerebral ventricles, while flexible endoscopes allow access to more remote or curved areas of the brain or spinal column.

Surgical approaches: Endoscopic procedures can be performed through natural holes in the body, such as the nostrils, or through small incisions made in the skull or spinal column.

Navigation and visualisation: Thanks to miniature cameras and advanced navigation systems, neurosurgeons can obtain clear images of target areas and navigate with precision.

2. Advantages of neuroendoscopy :

Minimally invasive: One of the main advantages of neuroendoscopy is its minimally invasive nature. This means smaller incisions, less damage to surrounding tissue and, as a result, faster recovery and less pain for the patient.

Improved visualisation: Endoscopy allows direct visualisation of brain structures, providing a detailed view that can surpass that of traditional imaging techniques.

- **Risk reduction**: By avoiding large cranial flaps and minimising manipulation of brain tissue, neuroendoscopy can reduce the risk of complications associated with more invasive procedures.
- **Reduced hospital stay**: Thanks to smaller incisions and faster recovery, patients can often leave hospital sooner than with traditional surgery.
- **Varied applications**: Neuroendoscopy is used to treat a variety of conditions, from brain tumours to hydrocephalus, cysts and some forms of brain haemorrhage.

Neuroendoscopy represents the intersection of advanced medical technology and the surgical art. It offers an alternative to traditional methods, enabling clinical challenges to be tackled with greater precision and delicacy. However, its success depends not only on the surgeon's mastery of the techniques, but also on close collaboration between the nurse, the surgeon and the entire medical team to ensure the patient's safety and well-being.

Interventional radiology : procedures and the role of the nurse

Interventional radiology (IR) is a fast-growing speciality that uses imaging to guide minimally invasive procedures for diagnostic or therapeutic purposes. Nurses play a vital role in this field, providing both direct patient care and close collaboration with interventional radiologists.

1. The main interventional radiology procedures :
- **Angiography and angioplasty**: Used to visualise and treat vascular problems such as occlusions or aneurysms.

Imaging-guided biopsies: Tissue samples are taken using imaging techniques for a precise diagnosis.

Embolisation: Used to stop bleeding or to block the blood supply to a tumour.

Radiofrequency ablation: Elimination of tumours using heat produced by radio waves.

Drainage: Insertion of a tube to drain accumulated fluids, such as abscesses.

2. Role of the interventional radiology nurse :

Pre-procedural assessment: Nurses assess the patient's state of health, medical history and medication, and identify any risk factors. They may also carry out preliminary tests, such as blood tests.

Preparing the patient: Informing the patient about the procedure, obtaining consents, placing the patient on the operating table, and ensuring sterilisation of the operating site.

Support during the procedure: Nurses monitor the patient's vital signs, administer medication or sedation if necessary, and interact with the radiologist to report any abnormalities or changes.

Post-procedure care: After the procedure, nurses monitor patients for possible complications, manage pain, assess incision or puncture sites, and provide instructions for returning home.

Education and communication: Nurses provide essential information to patients and their families, answer their questions and reassure them.

Interprofessional collaboration: Nurses work closely with radiologists, radiology technologists, anaesthetists and other members of the medical team to ensure optimal care.

Radiation protection management: Due to regular exposure to X-rays, IR nurses must be well informed about the principles of radiation protection and ensure their own safety as well as that of patients.

Interventional radiology combines medical imaging expertise with minimally invasive surgical techniques, enabling more targeted and often less traumatic treatments for the patient. The role of the nurse in this field is crucial, ensuring that every stage of the procedure is carried out safely and efficiently, while providing a positive experience for the patient.

Chapter 12:
SPECIFIC PHARMACOLOGY
NEUROSURGERY

Commonly used medicines
in neurosurgery and their effects

As a cutting-edge speciality, neurosurgery requires a specific range of drugs that not only help to manage pain, prevent infection and reduce inflammation, but also modulate neurological function during and after surgery. Here is a non-exhaustive list of drugs commonly used in neurosurgery and their associated effects:

1. Analgesics:
   - **Paracetamol (Acetaminophen)**: Often used for mild to moderate pain and fever.
   - **Opiates (Morphine, Fentanyl, Oxycontin)**: Prescribed to manage moderate to severe pain. These drugs can cause drowsiness, constipation and respiratory depression if used in excess.
2. Anti-inflammatories:
   - **Dexamethasone: A** potent corticosteroid often used to reduce cerebral oedema.
   - **Ibuprofen and Naproxen**: Non-steroidal anti-inflammatory drugs (NSAIDs) used for pain and inflammation. They may increase the risk of bleeding.
3. Anticonvulsants:
   - **Phenytoin (Dilantin), Carbamazepine (Tegretol), and Levetiracetam (Keppra)**: Used to prevent or treat epileptic seizures that may occur after brain surgery.

4. Osmotic agents:
   Mannitol: Used to reduce intracranial pressure in cases of cerebral oedema.
5. Diuretics:
   Furosemide (Lasix): Used to eliminate excess fluid and prevent or treat oedema.
6. Antibiotics:
   Various drugs, such as **Cefazolin**, can be administered prophylactically to prevent post-operative infections.
7. Muscle relaxation agents:
   Baclofen: Used to treat spasticity associated with conditions such as multiple sclerosis or after spinal cord surgery.
8. Anaesthetic agents:
   Medications such as **Propofol, Etomidate and Sevoflurane** are used to induce and maintain anaesthesia during surgery.
9. Blood pressure medication:
   Drugs such as **beta-blockers, alpha-agonists and vasodilators are** used to maintain stable blood pressure during surgery.
10. Anticoagulants and antiplatelets:
    Like **Heparin** or **Clopidogrel**, they are often used after certain operations to prevent the formation of clots.

Each of these drugs has its own range of side effects, interactions and contraindications. A thorough knowledge of these drugs, their mechanisms of action and their potential implications is essential for the neurosurgical nurse. Effective communication with patients about these drugs, their benefits and potential risks, is also crucial.

Drug interaction and implications for nurses

A drug interaction occurs when the effect or half-life of one drug is altered by taking another drug. These interactions may potentiate or attenuate the efficacy of the drugs, or even lead to new adverse reactions. For the neurosurgical nurse, understanding and monitoring these interactions is essential to ensure patient safety and effective treatment.

1. Implications for assessment:
Nurses must systematically take a full medication history of the patient, including prescription and over-the-counter medicines, supplements and herbal remedies. Nurses must also be aware of the indications for each drug, its dosage, frequency of administration and mechanism of action.

2. Implications for drug administration:
Nurses must be aware of the potential interactions between the drugs prescribed and those that the patient may already be taking. Some drugs, when administered together, may require a change in dosage or time of administration to minimise the risk of interaction.

3. Implications for surveillance:
Following drug administration, the nurse must monitor the patient for any signs or symptoms of drug interaction, such as increased toxicity, reduced efficacy or new adverse reactions. Monitoring of vital signs, clinical symptoms and, in some cases, serum drug levels is essential.

4. Implications for patient education:
Nurses have a crucial role to play in educating patients and their families about the risks of drug interactions, by encouraging them to always inform their healthcare professionals of all the medicines they are taking. It is also essential to inform patients of the potential signs and symptoms of drug interactions.

5. Implications for documentation:
The nurse must accurately document all drugs administered, as well as any reactions or concerns about potential interactions. If a drug interaction is suspected or identified, it should be reported to the medical team and documented in the patient's medical record.

6. Implications for collaboration:
Nurses need to work closely with pharmacists, doctors and other members of the healthcare team to manage drug interactions. Pharmacists, in particular, are an invaluable resource for identifying and managing drug interactions.

Drug interaction is a major concern in neurosurgery, as many patients may be on several drugs at the same time, each with its own implications and mechanisms of action. Vigilance, knowledge and proactive communication are essential to manage these interactions and ensure patient safety.

Managing anticoagulant and anti-epileptic drugs

In neurosurgery, drug management plays a crucial role in ensuring optimal patient outcomes. Among the commonly used drugs, anticoagulants and anti-epileptics occupy a central place, each with its own challenges and implications. Proper management of these drugs is essential to prevent potentially serious complications.

1. Anticoagulant drugs:
Anticoagulants, as their name suggests, are drugs that prevent blood clotting. They are often prescribed to treat or prevent thrombosis.

Use in neurosurgery: After certain neurosurgical procedures, there is an increased risk of blood clots forming. Anticoagulants may be administered to minimise this risk.

Associated challenges: The administration of anticoagulants must be carefully balanced. Excessive anticoagulation can lead to bleeding, while insufficient anticoagulation may not offer adequate protection against clot formation.

Monitoring: Patients on anticoagulants require regular monitoring of blood coagulation parameters. Nurses should be alert to any signs of bleeding, such as bruising, bleeding gums or black Feces.

2. Anti-epileptic drugs:
Anti-epileptic drugs are used to treat and prevent epileptic seizures. These drugs work by altering the electrical activity of the brain.

Use in neurosurgery: Patients undergoing neurosurgical procedures, particularly on the brain, may be at risk of post-operative seizures. Antiepileptic drugs may be given prophylactically or in response to a seizure.

Associated challenges: Monitoring blood levels of anti-epileptic drugs is essential to ensure that the patient is within the desired therapeutic range. Too little medication may not effectively control seizures, while too much may cause toxic side effects.

Monitoring: The nurse should watch for signs of toxicity from anti-epileptic drugs, such as drowsiness, dizziness or double vision. Particular attention should be paid to detecting any convulsive activity.

Implications for nurses:

Education: Nurses must educate patients and their families about the importance of taking medication regularly, potential side effects and the need for regular follow-up.

Coordination: Working closely with doctors, pharmacists and other health professionals, nurses play a key role in ensuring that these medicines are administered safely.

Documentation: All drug administration, side effects and adverse reactions must be carefully documented.

The management of anticoagulant and anti-epileptic drugs is an essential aspect of care in neurosurgery. With meticulous attention to detail and inter-professional collaboration, the nurse plays a central role in ensuring that these drugs offer maximum benefit while minimising the risks to the patient.

Chapter 13:
PAEDIATRIC PATIENTS
IN NEUROSURGERY

Anatomical features
and physiology in children

Childhood is a period of rapid growth and development, and as such has anatomical and physiological characteristics that are distinct from those of adults. These particularities influence the medical and surgical management of children, including in the field of neurosurgery.

1. The child's skull :
   Fontanelles: At birth, a child's skull is made up of several bones separated by soft spaces called fontanelles. These areas allow the skull to deform during birth and leave room for the rapid growth of the brain. They solidify over time, generally around the age of 2.
   Malleable skull: The flexibility of the child's skull allows a certain amount of expansion in the event of an increase in intracranial pressure. However, a prolonged increase in this pressure can lead to deformation.
2. The developing brain :
   Rapid growth: In the first few years of life, the brain undergoes rapid growth, almost doubling in size in the first year.
   Plasticity: Children's brains have a remarkable capacity to adapt. In the event of injury, other areas of the brain can often compensate for the lost function, a phenomenon less common in adults.

3. Spinal column and cord :

Flexibility: The child's spine is more flexible than the adult's, which influences the types of injury and deformity observed.

Growing spinal cord: The spinal cord in young children is proportionally longer than the spinal column, moving upwards with age. This must be taken into account during surgery.

4. Nervous system :

Myelination: Myelination, the process by which axons are covered with a myelin sheath, continues after birth, influencing the speed of nerve conduction.

Synaptogenesis: There is an explosion of synaptic formation in the first years of life, followed by a selective elimination of synapses, thus refining neuronal circuits.

5. Physiological responses :

Metabolism: Cerebral metabolism is higher in children than in adults, which means that children have higher energy requirements.

Response to medication: Drug metabolism, distribution and elimination may vary in children, necessitating dosage adjustments.

The anatomical and physiological differences between children and adults have major implications for healthcare professionals, particularly in neurosurgery. A thorough understanding of these particularities is essential to provide appropriate and effective care. For nurses working in paediatric neurosurgery, this knowledge enables them to adjust care, interpret signs and symptoms correctly, and work closely with the whole medical team to ensure the best possible outcome for the child.

Common paediatric neurosurgical conditions

Paediatrics presents a unique set of neurosurgical conditions that sometimes differ from those seen in adults. The management of these conditions requires specialist knowledge of the anatomical, physiological and developmental particularities of children. Here is an overview of these conditions.

1. Congenital malformations :

Hydrocephalus: Abnormal accumulation of cerebrospinal fluid in or around the brain. It may result from obstruction, reduced absorption or excessive production of fluid.

Spina bifida: A neural tube closure defect that can lead to protrusion of spinal cord structures through an opening in the spinal column.

Craniostenosis: Premature closure of the skull sutures, limiting the normal expansion of the brain as it grows.

2. Brain tumours :

Although less common than in adults, brain tumours are among the most common paediatric cancers. Common types include :

Medulloblastoma: A malignant tumour of the posterior fossa.

Pilocytic astrocytoma: A generally benign tumour that can be found anywhere in the brain.

Ependymoma: Tumour that develops from the ependymal cells that line the ventricles of the brain.

3. Craniocerebral trauma :

Children are particularly prone to falls and injuries, which can lead to varying degrees of head trauma.

4. Central nervous system infections :

Brain abscess: localised accumulation of pus in the brain following an infection.

Meningitis: Inflammation of the membranes surrounding the brain and spinal cord.

5. Epilepsy :

Some forms of epilepsy are specific to the paediatric population, such as West's syndrome or infantile spasms.

6. Vascular disorders :

Arteriovenous malformations (AVMs): Abnormal connections between arteries and veins, often present at birth.

Cavernomas: Vascular malformations that can cause bleeding or seizures.

7. Spinal cord anomalies :

Tethered cord syndrome: The spinal cord is abnormally attached to the spinal column, restricting its movement.

Paediatric neurosurgical care is a complex speciality, requiring a dedicated approach. For nurses working in this field, an in-depth knowledge of these conditions and their implications is essential in order to provide quality care, support families and collaborate effectively with the rest of the medical team.

The nurse's specific approach in relation to children and their families

In paediatric neurosurgery, the nurse is not just looking after one patient, but a dynamic whole, including the child and his or her family. The physiological, psychological and social needs of children differ from those of adults, and require a tailored, caring approach.

1. Age-appropriate communication :
   Using games: Incorporating games into the explanation of procedures can help to reduce children's anxiety.

   Simple language: Nurses will often have to simplify or adapt their explanations so that they are understandable to the child.
2. Creating a reassuring environment :
   Soothing atmosphere: Toys, bright colours or familiar elements can transform a hospital room into a less intimidating place.

   Parental presence: As far as possible, parents should be present during care to reassure the child.
3. Active involvement of parents :
   Parents can be trained in some basic care, enabling them to be actively involved in their child's recovery process.

   Recognition of parents as primary care partners is essential to ensure continuity of care.
4. Pain assessment :
   Pain in children can be expressed differently. Nurses must be trained to recognise these signs and to use pain scales adapted to children.

5. Holistic approach :
   Take into account the child's growth and development, and adapt care accordingly.

   Recognising and responding to children's emotional needs, which may vary according to their age and maturity.
6. Psychological support for the family :
   A child's illness or surgery is an upsetting ordeal for the whole family. Nurses must also support parents and siblings, offering them clear information and referring them to other professionals if necessary.

7. Therapeutic education :
    The nurse educates the family about the illness, post-operative care and rehabilitation. This education helps prepare the family for discharge from hospital.

Paediatric neurosurgery is a field in which the nurse plays a multidimensional role. In addition to clinical care, the nurse is an educator, emotional support and advocate for the child. Effective communication, compassion and a thorough understanding of the unique needs of the child and family are essential to providing quality care.

Chapter 14:
COMPLEMENTARY APPROACHES
IN NEUROSURGERY

Post-operative neurological rehabilitation

Post-operative neurological rehabilitation is a fundamental part of a patient's care after neurosurgery. It aims to restore, compensate for or adapt impaired functions, enabling the patient to regain a satisfactory level of autonomy and quality of life. This crucial phase requires interdisciplinary collaboration and the unfailing involvement of nurses.

1. Understanding the challenges of rehabilitation :
After neurosurgery, deficits may be motor, sensory or cognitive, or a combination of these. The main aim of rehabilitation is to enable patients to function as well as possible in their everyday environment.

2. Initial assessment :
Working with a rehabilitation team, the nurse assesses the patient's deficits, needs and goals. This assessment serves as the basis for drawing up an individualised rehabilitation plan.

3. Rehabilitation techniques :
- **Physiotherapy:** Focuses on motor recovery, coordination, muscle strength and balance.
- **Occupational therapy:** Helps patients to regain their everyday skills, adapting their environment and advising them on the use of technical aids.
- **Speech therapy:** Necessary in the event of language or swallowing disorders.

Neuropsychology: For patients with cognitive problems, sessions are aimed at working on memory, attention and executive functions.

4. The role of the nurse in rehabilitation :

Daily monitoring: Assessing progress, detecting any complications and adjusting care accordingly.

Education: informing patients and their families about exercise, the use of medication and any adaptations needed at home.

Psychological support: Rehabilitation can be a frustrating time for patients. The nurse plays a key role in providing emotional support.

Care coordination: Ensuring a smooth transition between hospital and home or rehabilitation centres.

5. The importance of interdisciplinarity :
Close collaboration between nurses, physiotherapists, occupational therapists, rehabilitation doctors, psychologists, social workers and other professionals is essential for comprehensive care.

6. Taking the family into account :
The family plays a crucial role in supporting and encouraging the patient. The nurse ensures that the family is well informed and involved in the process.

Post-operative neurological rehabilitation is a decisive stage that has a major influence on the patient's future. The nurse, through his or her constant presence and central role in care, is a pillar of this recovery phase, guaranteeing holistic care tailored to the patient's needs.

Alternative therapies : acupuncture, osteopathy, etc.

At the heart of the modern medical landscape lies a rich and diverse mix of traditional and alternative therapies. These therapies, although often marginal to conventional medical protocols, can offer significant additional benefits to neurosurgical patients. It is therefore vital for nurses to have an informed understanding of these therapies in order to guide and inform patients in the best possible way.

1. Acupuncture :

Originating in traditional Chinese medicine, acupuncture involves the insertion of fine needles into precise points on the body. These points are considered to be areas where energy, or "Qi", circulates.

Benefits in neurosurgery: Acupuncture can help manage post-operative pain, reduce inflammation and improve blood circulation.

The role of the nurse: to identify patients who could benefit from this approach, to know the right practitioners, and to integrate this care into the overall therapeutic plan.

2. Osteopathy:

This manual approach focuses on the detection, treatment and prevention of imbalances in the mobility of the body's tissues that can cause disorders.

Benefits in neurosurgery: Osteopathy can contribute to post-operative recovery by improving mobility and reducing musculoskeletal tension.

The nurse's role: To understand when osteopathy can be useful, to refer the patient to qualified osteopaths, and to ensure that this treatment is compatible with the patient's other care.

3. Other complementary therapies :

  Chiropractic: Focuses on the diagnosis, treatment and prevention of musculoskeletal disorders, particularly of the spine.

  Massage therapy: Massages can help relax muscles, improve circulation and reduce pain.

  Meditation and mindfulness: These practices can help patients manage the stress, pain and anxiety associated with their condition or procedure.

Although these alternative therapies do not replace traditional medical treatments, they can offer significant additional benefits for neurosurgical patients. The nurse, as the pivot of patient care, has a duty to be informed of these options, to ensure comprehensive and integrated management.

Method integration unconventional in the care plan

The advent of the era of integrative medicine constantly reminds us of the importance of considering the human being as a whole. The patient is not simply a sum of symptoms to be treated, but a complex entity whose needs go far beyond surgery or medication. Non-conventional methods, although sometimes disparaged, offer a holistic dimension to care, enabling a more complete approach to healing. As an essential link in the care chain, the neurosurgical nurse must be familiar with these methods and know how to integrate them judiciously.

1. Recognise the patient's individuality :
Each patient is unique, with his or her own beliefs, experiences and expectations. An effective care plan recognises this uniqueness and seeks to integrate it.

2. Understanding the different methods :

Homeopathy: Based on the principle of similarity, small doses are used to treat specific symptoms.

Phytotherapy: The use of plants for medicinal purposes, often in the form of infusions, decoctions or capsules.

Aromatherapy: The use of essential oils for a range of ailments, from pain to anxiety.

3. The importance of continuing education :

Nurses must keep abreast of the latest research and developments in unconventional therapies, in order to offer patients sound advice.

4. Collaboration with other professionals:

A network of qualified therapists (naturopaths, osteopaths, acupuncturists, etc.) enables nurses to direct patients to the best resources.

5. Assessment of specific patient needs :

Some patients may benefit more from complementary methods to manage pain, anxiety or other symptoms.

6. Integration into the care plan :

It is crucial to integrate these methods consistently. For example, if a patient is using herbal remedies, care must be taken to ensure that they do not interact negatively with the patient's medication.

7. Respect the patient's choices :

Some patients may be reluctant to use unconventional methods. It is essential to respect their choices, while providing objective information.

Integrating non-conventional methods into the care plan is a delicate exercise that requires knowledge, open-mindedness and discernment. The nurse, as an advocate for the patient's needs and rights, plays a central role in ensuring that this integration is carried out in an informed and beneficial way for the patient.

Chapter 15:
RESEARCH AND INNOVATION IN NEUROSURGERY

Latest advances and ongoing research

The field of neurosurgery, like many other medical fields, is constantly evolving. The intersection of technology, biology and medicine has led to advances that were once considered pure science fiction. In this sea of progress, it is essential for all healthcare professionals, particularly neurosurgical nurses, to stay informed and up to date.

1. Robot-assisted surgery:
Surgical robots offer greater precision, reduce human tremors and allow smaller incisions, resulting in faster recovery for patients. Systems such as the Da Vinci can already perform complex procedures with minimal invasiveness.

2. Advanced imaging:
The use of artificial intelligence and deep learning in medical imaging facilitates the detection and precise mapping of brain lesions. This enables more targeted and less invasive surgery.

3. Gene and cell therapy:
Research is underway to treat neurodegenerative diseases, such as Parkinson's disease or amyotrophic lateral sclerosis (ALS), by modifying genes or using stem cells.

4. Neuromodulation:
Using implants to modulate the brain's electrical activity has shown promise in treating conditions such as treatment-resistant depression, epilepsy and even some chronic pain.

5. 3D bioprinting:
The ability to 3D print biological tissue paves the way for the creation of personalised grafts to repair neurological damage.

6. Brain-machine interfaces:
Research into the creation of direct interfaces between the brain and machines could, in the future, help paralysed patients to regain certain functions or to communicate.

7. Laser microsurgery:
Using lasers to perform delicate procedures minimises damage to surrounding tissue and speeds healing.

8. Biomaterials research:
The development of new brain-compatible materials can reduce the risk of infection, rejection or inflammation after surgery.

The frontier of neurosurgery is constantly expanding thanks to technological innovations and extensive research. For the neurosurgical nurse, understanding these advances and how they can be applied clinically is essential to providing optimal care. However, it is also important to keep medical ethics in mind and ensure that each new method is applied in a way that is in the best interests of the patient.

Involvement of the nurse clinical research

Clinical research, which encompasses a range of activities from preliminary studies to phase IV clinical trials, is at the heart of medical advances. It enables us to understand diseases, develop new treatments and improve the quality of care. Nurses, with their unique proximity to patients and their in-depth understanding of the administration of care, play a crucial role in this process.

1. The nurse as a link between the patient and the research team :
The relationship of trust established between the nurse and the patient facilitates communication. The nurse is often the first point of contact for patients taking part in clinical studies, answering their questions, allaying their fears and ensuring that they understand and give informed consent.

2. Management of clinical assessments :
Nurses are often responsible for collecting data as part of clinical trials, whether through blood sampling, vital measurements, neurological assessments or other relevant tests.

3. Monitoring side effects and adverse reactions :
The nurse plays a crucial role in monitoring and documenting the side effects of study treatments. This careful monitoring can help to identify any potential problems quickly, thereby ensuring the safety of participants.

4. Education and training:
The nurse is often responsible for educating patients on the conduct of the trial, the protocols to be followed and the importance of compliance. In addition, the nurse may be called upon to train other members of staff on the specifics of the clinical trial.

5. Multidisciplinary collaboration:
By working closely with researchers, doctors, pharmacists and other healthcare professionals, the nurse helps to ensure that the trial is conducted in accordance with ethical and regulatory standards.

6. Active participation in research design:
Drawing on their clinical experience, nurses can offer valuable insights when designing studies, suggesting methodologies that take into account both science and the best patient experience.

7. Promotion of clinical research:
Nurses can act as advocates for clinical research within the medical community and the general public, raising

awareness of the benefits of clinical trials and encouraging participation.

Nurses' involvement in clinical research strengthens the bridge between clinical care and research. With their sensitivity to patients' needs and their clinical expertise, nurses are essential in ensuring that research is not only scientifically rigorous, but also ethical and patient-centred.

The future of neurosurgery : robotics, artificial intelligence, etc.

Neurosurgery, like many other medical disciplines, is constantly evolving. With the technological explosion of recent decades, we are on the cusp of a revolution in the way neurosurgical procedures are performed and envisaged. Advances in robotics, artificial intelligence (AI) and new technologies promise more precise, safer and effective interventions.

1. Robotics in neurosurgery :
Surgical robots, such as the famous da Vinci robot, have already changed the game in several surgical fields. In neurosurgery, these robots promise microscopic precision, minimising the risk of damaging healthy tissue. They can be programmed to perform repetitive tasks with unrivalled accuracy, while allowing the surgeon to control the operation at every stage.

2. Artificial intelligence and neuroimaging:
AI has the potential to transform neuroimaging. Sophisticated algorithms can help to quickly identify abnormalities, predict the risk of certain conditions or even guide surgeons in real time during surgery. What's more, with machine learning, these systems can continually improve by analysing large amounts of data.

3. Augmented reality and virtual reality:

These technologies give neurosurgeons a three-dimensional view of the patient's brain or spine, enabling more precise surgical planning. During surgery, surgeons can 'see' the area they are operating on superimposed on digital images, providing better guidance and reducing risks.

4. Nanotechnology:

Nanoparticles could be used to deliver drugs directly to specific areas of the brain, offering targeted treatment for conditions such as brain tumours. This could reduce the side effects associated with traditional chemotherapy.

5. Brain-machine interface :

These interfaces, which enable direct communication between the brain and an external device, could revolutionise the treatment of spinal cord injuries, neurodegenerative diseases and other conditions. Imagine a paralysed patient who can control an exoskeleton using his or her thoughts!

6. Training and education with AI:

AI-based systems can also play a role in training future neurosurgeons, offering realistic simulations and adaptive learning scenarios.

The future of neurosurgery is bright, with a convergence of technologies offering new ways of treating, diagnosing and approaching neurological conditions. However, with these advances comes the need for ongoing training, rigorous ethics and constant consideration of the humanity behind every diagnosis. Technology may evolve, but the heart of medicine remains the patient's well-being.

Chapter 16:
PREVENTION AND PATIENT EDUCATION

Preventive education to reduce the risk of neurological diseases

Preventive education, focusing on raising public awareness of healthy behaviours and taking proactive measures, is a powerful tool for reducing the risk of neurological diseases. Preventing diseases, particularly those affecting the nervous system, can not only improve quality of life but also reduce the economic and emotional burden for individuals, their families and society as a whole.

1. Raising awareness of head injuries :
Head injuries, whether minor or serious, can have long-term consequences for neurological health. Education on the importance of wearing a helmet when taking part in high-risk sports or activities, and on road safety measures, is crucial.

2. Promoting healthy eating:
Numerous studies have shown that what we eat can influence our brain health. A balanced diet rich in antioxidants, omega-3s and essential nutrients can help prevent conditions such as dementia and Alzheimer's disease.

3. The importance of physical activity:
Regular exercise stimulates blood circulation, which can help prevent strokes and other neurological conditions. Physical activity has also been associated with a reduced risk of cognitive decline.

4. Stress management :
Chronic stress can have detrimental effects on the brain. Education on relaxation techniques, such as meditation,

yoga and deep breathing, can be beneficial for mental and neurological health.

5. Avoid harmful substances:
Raising awareness of the dangers of excessive alcohol consumption, drug use and exposure to certain environmental toxins can help prevent their negative impact on the nervous system.

6. Regular control of blood pressure and diabetes
These two factors are closely linked to neurological health. High blood pressure and uncontrolled diabetes can damage the blood vessels in the brain, increasing the risk of stroke and dementia.

7. Promoting restful sleep :
Quality sleep is essential for brain regeneration and memory consolidation. Educating people about the importance of sleep and methods of improving sleep quality can have a significant impact on the prevention of neurological diseases.

8. Vaccination :
Some infections can lead to neurological complications. Raising awareness of the importance of vaccination against diseases such as meningitis, rabies and Japanese encephalitis is therefore crucial.

9. Mental health promotion:
Conditions such as depression, anxiety or bipolar disorder can have neurological implications. It is essential to educate the public about recognising signs and symptoms and the importance of appropriate management.

Preventive education is a powerful way of promoting the health and well-being of the population. By raising awareness and equipping individuals to make informed decisions about their health, we can reduce the incidence of neurological diseases and improve the quality of life.

Education strategies to improve post-operative compliance

Ensuring patients' post-operative compliance is an essential part of optimising surgical outcomes and minimising potential complications. Compliance, i.e. adherence to medical recommendations, is often a challenge due to the complexity of guidelines, patient fears or misconceptions, and various other barriers. Patient education is therefore a key strategy for improving compliance. Let's take a look at some effective education strategies.

1. Assessment of individual needs :
Every patient is unique. Understanding their needs, concerns and level of knowledge is the starting point. Use questionnaires or interviews to assess these elements.

2. Use of suitable teaching materials :
Leaflets, videos, anatomical models and mobile apps can be used to provide information. Make sure these materials are up to date, clear and understandable to the patient.

3. Individual and group education sessions:
While individual sessions provide personalised attention, group sessions can offer peer-to-peer interaction and support.

4. Practical demonstrations:
For example, show patients how to clean an incision or how to perform certain physiotherapy exercises. Seeing and doing can improve understanding and confidence.

5. Involvement of family and carers :
Often it is family members or carers who will support the patient at home. Involving them in the educational process can reinforce compliance.

6. Reminders and follow-ups:
Phone calls, text messages or apps can be used to remind patients of their medication, appointments or other important instructions.

7. Provide written information:
Oral instructions are easily forgotten. Providing a written summary of post-operative instructions can help patients to refer back to the recommendations.

8. Encourage a questioning environment:
Encourage patients to ask questions. The more they understand their situation, the more likely they are to comply with the recommendations.

9. Review sessions:
Organise follow-up sessions to review post-operative instructions, clarify doubts and reinforce desired behaviours.

10. Patient feedback:
Solicit feedback on educational materials and sessions to continue to improve and refine approaches.

11. Reinforcement of benefits :
Explain clearly to the patient why each directive is important and how it contributes to their recovery.

12. Create a helpline:
Provide a helpline or a way for patients to ask questions or report problems between appointments. Knowing they have ongoing support can increase compliance.

Education is a powerful tool for improving post-operative compliance. By adopting a multi-dimensional, patient-centred approach and adapting to individual needs, healthcare professionals can optimise surgical outcomes and ensure that patients receive the best possible care after surgery.

Use of digital tools for patient education

In a world where technology plays an increasingly dominant role, harnessing digital tools for patient education is becoming not only relevant, but essential. These tools offer a variety of ways to improve patient understanding, compliance and engagement.

1. Dedicated mobile applications :
Many applications are designed specifically to provide medical information, monitor patient progress, remind patients of medication or appointments, and offer advice on managing certain conditions. These applications can be customised to meet the specific needs of each patient.

2. Online learning platforms:
There are dedicated platforms where patients can follow learning modules, explanatory videos and participate in discussion forums. These platforms offer an interactive learning experience.

3. Virtual and augmented reality:
These immersive technologies can help patients visualise complex processes, understand their anatomy or how a treatment works. For example, visualising surgery or understanding the process of repairing a fracture.

4. Patient portals:
Secure portals where patients can access their medical records, book appointments, ask questions and receive answers from their medical team, or track their progress.

5. Webinars and online sessions:
Video conferencing platforms make it possible to organise education sessions for large groups of patients, where they can interact with healthcare professionals and ask questions in real time.

6. Medical chatbots:
Chatbots programmed to provide answers to common medical questions, guide patients or even make an initial diagnosis based on the symptoms described.

7. Educational videos:
Videos, accessible via YouTube or other platforms, can illustrate concepts, procedures or advice for patients. They offer a visual learning method that can be more engaging.

8. Self-assessment tools:
Online questionnaires or quizzes that allow patients to assess their knowledge, reinforce what they have learned and identify areas where they may need further education.

9. Reminders and notifications :
Push alerts or text messages can remind patients of essential information, appointments or medicines to take.
10. Social networks:
Patient groups on platforms such as Facebook or LinkedIn can provide a space to share experiences, ask questions and receive information.

The integration of digital tools in patient education does not replace human interaction, but complements and enriches it. With the constant advent of new technologies and the ability to adapt these tools to patients' needs, healthcare professionals have a growing arsenal at their disposal to optimise patient education and engagement. When used judiciously, these tools have the potential to significantly improve patient care and outcomes.

Chapter 17:
HOSPITAL-ACQUIRED INFECTIONS IN NEUROSURGERY

Understanding the sources of infection

Infections are caused by pathogens such as bacteria, viruses, fungi and parasites. To prevent infections effectively, particularly in a medical environment, it is crucial to understand their sources and modes of transmission. Let's delve into this microscopic world together.

1. Bacteria :
These single-celled micro-organisms can live in almost any environment, from the bottom of the ocean to inside the human body. While many are beneficial to us, some can cause disease, such as staphylococcus aureus, which causes skin infections, or Koch's bacillus, which causes tuberculosis.

2. Viruses :
Smaller than bacteria, viruses can only reproduce inside the cells of other organisms. These may be animals, plants or humans. Examples include HIV, the influenza virus and SARS-CoV-2, which causes COVID-19.

3. Fungi:
Although they are essential for breaking down organic matter, some fungi can cause infections, particularly on the skin, such as mycosis, or the lungs, such as Pneumocystis pneumonia.

4. Parasites :
These organisms live and feed on other living things. Common parasitic diseases include malaria, giardiasis and toxoplasmosis.

Sources of infection :

- **Direct contact:** Pathogens can be transmitted by physical contact, such as shaking hands, kissing or biting.
- **Droplet transmission:** Coughs and sneezes release droplets containing pathogens that can infect other people if they inhale these droplets.
- **Food and water:** Eating or drinking contaminated products can lead to infections. Examples: salmonella, hepatitis A.
- **Contact with an infected surface:** Touching a contaminated surface and then touching your mouth, eyes or nose can lead to infection.
- **Vector-borne transmission:** Some pathogens are transmitted by insects. The mosquito is the vector of malaria, for example.
- **Animal transmission:** Animals can carry pathogens that can infect humans, such as the rabies virus.
- **Airborne transmission:** In rare cases, pathogens can be released into the air and breathed in. Tuberculosis can spread in this way.

Prevention :

- **Personal hygiene:** Regular hand washing is essential.
- **Vaccination: A** preventive method against certain infections.
- **Food safety:** Cook properly and avoid cross-contamination.
- **Protection against mosquitoes:** Use of mosquito nets or repellents.
- **Wearing protective equipment:** In a medical setting, wearing masks, gloves and gowns can reduce the spread of the disease.

Understanding the sources of infection is the first step in preventing their spread. In the medical field, this understanding is the cornerstone of effective prevention and rapid response to infectious disease outbreaks.

Prevention protocols and intervention

In the world of medicine, prevention and intervention are two sides of the same coin. Prevention aims to prevent an undesirable event from occurring, while intervention enables rapid and effective action to be taken in the event of an unforeseen event. Protocols are established to ensure that each step is carried out consistently, thereby reducing risk and maximising safety.

Prevention :
1. Hand hygiene :
   - Systematic hand washing before and after any contact with a patient, using soap and water or a hydro-alcoholic solution.
   - Regular staff training in appropriate techniques.
2. Use of personal protective equipment (PPE) :
   - Choosing the right PPE for the job: gloves, masks, goggles, smocks, etc.
   - Training in the correct fitting, removal and disposal of PPE.
3. Medical waste management :
   - Appropriate classification, disposal and disinfection of waste.
   - Staff training in safe waste handling.
4. Vaccination :
   - Ensure that staff are up to date with their vaccinations, including against hepatitis B, influenza and other relevant diseases.
   - Advice on vaccinating patients, where appropriate.
5. Further training :
   - Regular training sessions and updates for staff on the latest recommendations and techniques.
Speech:
1. Quick identification :
   - Protocols for rapidly recognising the signs and symptoms of an infection or other complication.

Triage tools to prioritise interventions.
2. Isolation :
Setting up isolation zones for patients showing symptoms of highly contagious infections.
Staff training on the admission, management and discharge of patients in isolation.
3. Processing :
Clearly defined drug protocols depending on the diagnosis.
Multidisciplinary approach with collaboration between different specialists where necessary.
4. Reporting :
Notification of nosocomial infections or outbreaks to the administration and public health authorities, if necessary.
Monitoring systems to identify underlying causes and prevent recurrences.
5. Review and improvement :
Regular evaluation of incidents and interventions to improve protocols.
Feedback and sharing of lessons learned with all staff.

The rigorous implementation of prevention and intervention protocols is crucial to ensuring the safety of patients and staff. These protocols require regular updating based on the latest research and ongoing training to ensure that every member of the team is equipped to provide the best possible care.

The crucial role of the nurse in the prevention of infections

Infection prevention is one of the cornerstones of nursing practice. Beyond simple medical care, nurses play a fundamental role in ensuring the safety and well-being of patients. In the world of neurosurgery, where patients can be particularly vulnerable to infection due to invasive procedures, the role of the nurse is all the more essential.

1. The first line of defence :
Nurses are often the first healthcare professionals to interact directly with patients, making them sentinels in the early detection of signs of infection. A simple physical examination, observation of the skin or wounds, or even measuring the temperature, can alert you to a possible infection.

2. Impeccable hygiene :
The importance of hand washing cannot be underestimated. By this simple action, nurses considerably reduce the risk of transmitting pathogens. What's more, by setting an example, they also encourage patients, their relatives and other members of the medical team to adopt rigorous hygiene.

3. Wound management :
Neurosurgical operations can result in major wounds. The nurse ensures that these are cleaned and aseptic, and monitors for any signs of infection. They also ensure that prophylactic antibiotics are properly administered where necessary.

4. Patient and family education :
By informing patients and their families about the signs of infection and preventive measures, nurses create an alliance to reinforce vigilance. This education enables rapid detection and treatment if an infection develops.

5. Working with the medical team :
The nurse is the link between the patient and the rest of the medical team. By effectively communicating any signs of infection or identified risks, they facilitate rapid and appropriate intervention.

6. Controlling medical devices :
Catheters, drains, probes and other devices can be entry points for infections. Nurses ensure that they are handled

aseptically, maintained and replaced in accordance with established protocols.

7. Participation in the development of protocols :

With their bedside experience, nurses are often best placed to recommend improvements or adjustments to existing infection control protocols.

8. Continuing education :

Nurses must keep up to date with the latest discoveries and recommendations in infection prevention. This enables them to adjust their practice and reinforce their role as patient protectors.

Far from being mere operatives, nurses are key players in the prevention of infections, particularly in neurosurgery. Their proactive role, expertise and proximity to patients make them key players in the safety and quality of care.

Chapter 18:
ETHICS AT THE END OF LIFE
IN NEUROSURGERY

Decision-making at the end of life
for neurosurgical patients

End-of-life decision-making for neurosurgical patients is an emotional and ethical journey, intertwined with a multitude of medical, personal and societal considerations. This complexity is accentuated by the unique and mysterious nature of the brain, the organ that shapes our identity, our memories and our desires, and which lies at the heart of neurosurgical interventions.

Patients faced with serious neurosurgical conditions, whether aggressive brain tumours, traumatic injuries or advanced neurodegenerative diseases, can be faced with agonising decisions. When disease alters the brain, it often calls into question not only the viability of life, but also its quality, the meaning of existence and the very essence of what makes us human.

These decisions are not taken lightly and require a holistic, patient-centred approach. Although neurosurgeons have technical expertise, they recognise the importance of involving the patient, the family and often a multidisciplinary team in the decision-making process. These teams may include neurologists, specialist nurses, psychologists, chaplains and social workers, all united to navigate these tumultuous waters.
The questions addressed are profound: When is it appropriate to consider withdrawing life support? What role

do advance directives play, and how can we ensure that they accurately reflect the patient's wishes?

How can we manage pain and discomfort while respecting the patient's wishes? And beyond medicalisation, how can we help patients and families to find meaning, closure or even hope in these darkest of moments?

Another challenge lies in respecting cultural and spiritual beliefs, as these can have a profound influence on end-of-life decisions. Open, empathetic and respectful communication is therefore essential to build trust and to understand and honour the wishes of patients and their families.

End-of-life decision-making for neurosurgical patients goes far beyond medicine. It is an exploration of the depths of humanity, values and beliefs. It is a reminder that, even in the darkest moments, every decision, every action, must be guided by compassion, respect and integrity.

The role of the nurse
in palliative care in neurosurgery

Palliative care, which focuses on pain relief and patient well-being rather than cure, is of vital importance in neurosurgery. In this context, the nurse plays a pivotal role. While the neurosurgeon concentrates on specific interventions to the brain or spinal cord, the nurse provides comprehensive, holistic and ongoing care for the patient, both physically and emotionally.

From the moment of diagnosis, the nurse is often the first person patients and their families turn to for answers, support and guidance. They are the guardians of their well-being, ensuring that their symptoms are managed effectively and that they receive clear and understandable information.

On the physical side, the neurosurgical nurse specialises in pain management, which can be particularly complex in these patients. This may involve a combination of medication, relaxation techniques and other interventions to ensure patient comfort.

But the role of the nurse goes far beyond the physical aspects. The nature of neurosurgical conditions can often have profound emotional and psychological consequences. Patients may be faced with cognitive deficits or personality changes, or they may be mourning the loss of their former lives. The nurse is there to support them through these challenges, offering a listening ear, a shoulder to cry on and advice on navigating these troubled waters.

Nurses also work closely with a palliative care team, made up of other healthcare professionals, to develop a care plan tailored to each patient. This may include sessions with psychologists, chaplains, social workers and other therapists to ensure comprehensive care.

The nurse is also a pillar of support for the patient's family. At difficult times, the family may feel lost, overwhelmed or powerless in the face of their loved one's illness. The nurse guides them through the process, helps them understand what to expect and supports them in their own grieving process.

The neurosurgical nurse working in palliative care is much more than a simple provider of medical care. They are the beating heart of the care team, bringing humanity, compassion and expertise to a situation that might otherwise seem insurmountable. In the darkest moments, the nurse reminds everyone that every day, every moment, has value and deserves to be lived to the full.

Sensitive communication with families

Communication with the families of neurosurgical patients is of fundamental importance. It must be marked by particular sensitivity and empathy, as these families are faced with realities that are often complex, sometimes frightening and always emotionally charged. The nurse, as the essential bridge between the patient, the medical team and the relatives, is ideally placed to take on this communication role.

First, it's important to recognise that every family is unique. Each member has their own feelings, fears, hopes and concerns. Understanding these dynamics enables nurses to adapt and personalise their communication. This requires active listening, where the nurse is fully present, without judgement, to hear and understand the family's needs.

The choice of words is also crucial. Medical terms, although familiar to the nurse, can be foreign and intimidating to the family. They need to be simplified without minimising or devaluing the information, to make the message clear and understandable. Metaphors and analogies can often help to clarify complicated concepts.

It is also essential to encourage questions. Families may be reluctant to ask questions for fear of appearing ignorant or annoying the medical staff. By creating a welcoming environment and openly inviting questions, the nurse can allay these fears and ensure that the family feels informed and supported.

But beyond words, non-verbal communication plays an equally important role. A simple reassuring touch, eye contact or patient listening can convey as much, if not more, than words. These gestures show the family that they are valued and taken into consideration.

It is also essential to recognise and respect the family's decisions, even if they differ from medical opinions or recommendations. Autonomy and respect for the dignity of each individual must be at the heart of nursing practice.

Finally, it is important to recognise the importance of emotional support. Families of neurosurgical patients can experience a range of emotions from fear and anger to denial and guilt. Nurses, through their experience and training, are able to provide emotional support, whether by offering a shoulder to cry on, providing resources or simply being present.

Sensitive communication with families is a delicate art, requiring patience, empathy and skill. But when done well, it can make a profound difference to a family's experience, transforming a potentially traumatic period into a journey of healing and hope.

Chapter 19:
THE IMPACT OF TELEMEDICINE IN NEUROSURGERY

Use of technology for remote consultations

In an increasingly interconnected world, technological advances have created unprecedented opportunities for medical care. One of the most remarkable innovations of recent years is the ability to carry out consultations at a distance, using a variety of technological tools. This mode of consultation, sometimes referred to as telemedicine, makes it possible to improve access to care, reduce costs and provide specialised services, even in remote areas.

The magic of connection
Using secure videoconferencing platforms, nurses and patients can see each other and communicate in real time, despite the distance that separates them. It's not just an audio conversation: the visual can be used to observe clinical signs, assess the patient's emotional state and establish a deeper connection. In addition, connected devices can transmit vital data, such as blood pressure or heart rate, directly to the nurse during the consultation.

Equal access to healthcare
Telemedicine breaks down geographical barriers. For patients living in rural or remote areas, or those who find it difficult to travel, the possibility of having a consultation at a distance is a real boon. They can access specialist care, such as neurosurgery, without having to travel long distances.

Save time and cut costs
Remote consultations reduce the need for travel, which means time savings for patients and healthcare professionals. They can also help reduce the costs associated with travel, accommodation or even face-to-face consultations.

Necessary precautions
However, telemedicine is not without its challenges. It is crucial to guarantee the confidentiality and security of patient data. The platforms used must comply with current data protection regulations. It is also important to ensure that nurses are properly trained in the use of these technologies, and to have a contingency plan in place in the event of technological failure.

Towards a connected future
Remote consultations are likely to be the future of many medical specialities, including neurosurgery. As technology evolves and new innovations emerge, it is essential that healthcare professionals, and nurses in particular, remain at the forefront of these changes. Embracing technology while preserving the human aspect of care is the challenge that telemedicine offers. And in the face of this challenge, nurses, with their central role in patient care, have everything to gain.

Post-operative monitoring via digital platforms

The advent of digital technologies has revolutionised patient care, offering new ways of monitoring their post-operative condition. Digital platforms now make it possible to monitor patients in real time, even remotely, guaranteeing continuity of care, better follow-up and optimised post-operative results.

Customised, real-time monitoring

Using connected devices and specialised applications, vital patient parameters such as heart rate, blood pressure and temperature can be continuously monitored and transmitted to a centralised platform. Nurses and the entire care team can access this data in real time, enabling rapid intervention in the event of an anomaly or complication.

The importance of self-monitoring

These platforms also give patients the opportunity to become actively involved in their own follow-up. They can enter data such as pain, postoperative symptoms or even share photos of the surgical wound. This self-monitoring strengthens the patient-carer bond and encourages collaborative care.

Alerts in the event of complications

One of the main advantages of digital platforms is the ability to set up automated alerts. If a parameter falls outside pre-established limits, or if a patient reports a worrying symptom, the medical team is immediately alerted, enabling rapid action to be taken.

Security and confidentiality first and foremost

As with any health-related technology, data security is paramount. Platforms must guarantee the confidentiality of information, while ensuring reliable data transmission. Regulations, often strict, govern these systems to protect both patients and healthcare professionals.

A future focused on remote surveillance

Post-operative monitoring via digital platforms is set to develop further in the coming years. It offers an appropriate response to the current challenges in healthcare, where optimising resources and remote management are becoming increasingly important. However, it is essential to remember that these technologies, however advanced, do not replace the clinical judgement and expertise of healthcare professionals. They are there to complement and reinforce them and, ultimately, to guarantee the best possible care for each patient.

Implications for nurses :
benefits, challenges and training

With the rise of digital platforms in neurosurgery, nurses are at the forefront of this development, playing a pivotal role in integrating these tools into the care pathway. These new responsibilities, while offering many advantages, come with challenges and require appropriate training.

Advantages :

Continuity of care: thanks to real-time monitoring, nurses can ensure continuity of post-operative care, even when the patient is away from the hospital.

Time optimisation: Digital platforms enable information to be centralised, making it easier to monitor patients and detect complications at an early stage.

Improved communication: The platforms promote fluid communication between the various healthcare professionals and with the patients themselves.

Strengthening the role of the nurse: Thanks to these tools, nurses are positioned as key players in remote monitoring, reinforcing their central role in postoperative follow-up.

Challenges :

Data confidentiality : With the constant exchange of medical information, nurses need to be particularly vigilant about data protection.

Technological dependence: Although digital platforms are invaluable tools, they can also fail. It is therefore crucial not to rely on them blindly and to maintain clinical vigilance.

Resistance to change: The introduction of new tools can provoke resistance from both patients and carers.

Alert management: The proliferation of data can lead to a large number of alerts, some of which may be irrelevant.

Training required :

Mastery of digital tools: Nurses must be trained in the use of platforms, from their interface to data management.

Cybersecurity training: It is crucial that nurses are aware of data security issues and know the protocols to follow in the event of a breach.

Patient-centred approach: Beyond the technology, it is essential that the nurse remains focused on the patient, adapting remote monitoring to each individual situation.

Continuous updating: The field of digital health is evolving rapidly. Regular training and knowledge updates are necessary to stay at the cutting edge of this speciality.

While digital platforms in neurosurgery open up exciting new prospects, they also require nurses' skills and professional practices to evolve. Nurses, who are at the heart of this revolution, have everything to gain from embracing these changes, while remaining faithful to their primary mission: guaranteeing the well-being and safety of patients.

Chapter 20:
APPROACH MANAGEMENT AND IMPLANTABLE DEVICES

External ventricular drainage, drug pumps, stimulators

In neurosurgery, various medical devices are commonly used to improve patients' quality of life, treat certain pathologies or prevent complications. Among these, external ventricular drainage (EVD), drug pumps and stimulators stand out for their technical nature and crucial importance. Let's take a closer look at the role of these tools, their indications and the way nurses interact with them.

1. External ventricular drainage (EVD) :

   Main function: EVGs are used to drain excess cerebrospinal fluid (CSF) from the brain to an external pouch, often in cases of hydrocephalus or following surgery.

   Indications: They are commonly indicated in cases of high intracranial pressure, haemorrhage or infection.

   The nurse's role: monitoring flow, preventing infection, managing complications such as blocked drains or haemorrhage, and educating patients and their families about its use.

2. Medication pumps :

   Primary function: These devices deliver drugs directly to the target area, such as the spinal cord, providing targeted relief and reducing side effects.

   Indications: Commonly used to administer antispasmodics, analgesics or chemotherapeutic agents.

The nurse's role: To ensure that the pump is working properly, to monitor for signs of complications, to refill the medication, to educate the patient about its use and to monitor potential side effects.

3. Stimulators :

Main function: These devices deliver small electrical impulses to specific areas of the brain or nervous system to treat various conditions.

Indications: Used to treat Parkinson's disease, epilepsy, certain chronic pain conditions and other disorders.

The nurse's role: To ensure that the device is working properly, to help with programming, to educate the patient about how it works, to monitor the patient's responses and to ensure that the electrodes remain in place.

Each of these devices plays an essential role in neurosurgical treatment, helping to improve patients' quality of life and effectively treat their conditions. For nurses, understanding these tools, how they work and their implications is crucial to ensuring optimal care and patient safety.

Monitoring, maintenance and possible complications

The management of neurosurgical patients goes far beyond the simple operation. Once the patient is fitted with devices such as external ventricular drainage, drug pumps or stimulators, constant monitoring, regular maintenance and prevention of possible complications become an absolute priority.

1. Monitoring :

Main objective: To ensure that the device functions correctly and that the patient remains stable.

Key points for nurses :

Monitor vital signs regularly.

Observe any changes in the patient's behaviour or level of consciousness.

Check the flow rate of the EVGs, ensure that the fluid drained is clear and that there are no signs of infection.

Check the implant site for redness, swelling or oozing.

Monitoring doses and dispensing medication via pumps.

Assess the patient's effectiveness and response to the stimulators.

2. Maintenance :

Main objective: To guarantee the proper long-term operation of the devices and the health of the patient.

Key points for nurses :

Regularly clean the implant site in accordance with hospital protocols.

Recharge or replace device batteries if necessary.

Ensure regular replacement of medicines in the pumps.

Program or reprogram the stimulators according to the patient's needs.

Educating patients and their families about home care.

3. Possible complications :

Main objective: To quickly detect any problems and intervene to resolve them.

Key points for nurses :

Infections : The implant site may become infected. Look out for signs such as redness, heat, pain, oozing or fever.

- **Blockages or leaks:** DVEs can become blocked or leak, compromising their function.
- **Adverse reactions:** The medicines delivered by the pumps may cause side effects.
- **Device failure:** All devices can eventually fail or deprogram.
- **Unexpected responses:** Although beneficial, stimulators can sometimes cause strange sensations or involuntary movements.

Managing these devices requires special expertise. For nurses, this means not only having technical skills, but also knowing how to interpret the subtle signs of complications, anticipate problems before they arise and reassure patients throughout their journey. Regular monitoring and maintenance, combined with rapid intervention in the event of complications, are essential to ensure the success of neurosurgical treatment and patient safety.

Patient and family education on home management

When a neurosurgical patient is about to be discharged home, a smooth and efficient transition is essential to ensure the patient's safety and well-being. To achieve this, educating the patient and their family about managing care at home is a crucial step. The main objective is to ensure that the patient receives the appropriate care while enabling the family to feel competent and supported.

1. Understanding the condition :
It is essential that patients and their families understand the nature and severity of the condition, as well as the long-term implications. Illustrated brochures, videos or information sessions can be helpful.

2. Daily routine :

Patients and their families must be informed about basic activities, mobility and dietary restrictions. This also includes instructions on how to get out of bed, take a shower, do light exercise and manage pain.

3. Wound and device care :

Practical demonstrations on how to clean incisions, change dressings, monitor for signs of infection and maintain any implanted devices (e.g. pumps or stimulators) are essential.

4. Medication :

Patients need to know how, when and why to take their medication. They also need to know about possible side effects and what to look out for.

5. Symptom monitoring :

Educate on the early warning signs and symptoms of complications, such as changes in level of consciousness, severe headaches, nausea or sudden weakness.

6. Support services :

Provide information on available services such as support groups, rehabilitation, complementary therapies and telemedicine.

7. Adaptation strategies :

Offer resources on stress management, emotional support and methods of coping with the new normal, such as meditation or therapy.

8. Follow-up visits :

It is essential to stress the importance of follow-up appointments and to provide a clear calendar with the dates and contact details of the specialists.

9. Availability in case of emergency :

Patients and their families need to know who to contact in an emergency, especially outside normal office hours.

10. Resources and references :

Provide a list of recommended reading, trusted websites and relevant contacts for further information.

Patient and family education is an ongoing process that requires open communication, patience and empathy. A neurosurgical nurse plays a central role in acting as a link between the complex medical world and the day-to-day needs of the patient, ensuring that the patient and family feel equipped and confident to manage the challenges ahead.

Chapter 21:
TUMOUR PATHOLOGIES
IN NEUROSURGERY

Understanding the different types
Nervous system tumours

The nervous system, made up of the brain, spinal cord and nerves, is a complex network responsible for a multitude of bodily functions. Unfortunately, it is susceptible to a variety of tumours. These tumours can be benign (non-cancerous) or malignant (cancerous), and their origin, behaviour and treatment can vary considerably.

1. Primary versus metastatic tumours :
Primary tumours start in the nervous system itself, while metastatic tumours originate in other parts of the body and have spread to the brain or spinal cord.

2. Glial tumours (gliomas) :
  Astrocytomas: These form from astrocytes, the cells that support neurons. Glioblastomas are the most aggressive form of astrocytoma.
  Oligodendrogliomas: These originate from oligodendrocytes, the cells that surround and isolate neurons.
  Ependymomas: These develop from the ependymal cells that line the ventricles of the brain and the central canal of the spinal cord.

3. Neuronal tumours :
  Neuroblastomas: These are common in children and often develop in the adrenal glands.

Gangliogliomas: These are rare tumours which often form in the temporal lobe of the brain.

4. Meningeal tumours :
Meningiomas: These develop from the membranes surrounding the brain and spinal cord, known as the meninges. Although generally benign, they can exert pressure on the brain or spinal cord.

5. Tumours of the pituitary gland :
They form in the pituitary gland, a small gland at the base of the brain. Although generally benign, they can affect hormone production.

6. Nerve tumours :
Neurofibromas: These come from the cells surrounding the peripheral nerves. They are often associated with a genetic disease called neurofibromatosis.
Schwannomas: These are similar to neurofibromas but arise specifically from Schwann cells.

7. Pineal tumours :
They form in the pineal gland, a small gland in the brain responsible for producing melatonin.

8. Metastatic tumours :
They start in other parts of the body, such as the lung, breast, skin or elsewhere, and then spread to the brain.

Understanding tumours of the nervous system is essential for the diagnosis, management and treatment of these conditions. Although this list is not exhaustive, it provides an overview of common tumours affecting the nervous system. Early detection, appropriate management and effective communication between healthcare professionals and patients are crucial to optimising outcomes and quality of life for those affected.

Specific post-operative management neuro-oncology patients

The post-operative management of patients who have undergone surgery for a tumour of the nervous system represents a unique challenge, given the delicacy and complexity of this anatomical area. Neuro-oncology patients require special attention to ensure not only their physical recovery, but also their emotional well-being.

1. Neurological monitoring :
After neuro-oncological surgery, close neurological monitoring is essential. This includes regular checks on consciousness, muscle strength, sensitivity, reflexes and signs of elevated intracranial pressure.

2. Pain management :
Post-operative pain can be a major problem. It must be assessed frequently and treated appropriately with analgesics, while monitoring side effects.

3. Prevention of complications :
   Cerebral oedema: This can be reduced with medication such as corticosteroids.
   Haematomas: Monitoring bleeding is essential for the early detection of intracranial haematomas.
   Infections: Signs of infection, such as fever or redness around the surgical wound, must be quickly identified and treated.

4. Re-education and rehabilitation :
Depending on the location and size of the tumour, patients may require rehabilitation therapies such as physiotherapy, occupational therapy or speech therapy.

5. Emotional support :
The diagnosis of a brain tumour can be devastating for patients and their families. It is therefore essential to provide psychological support, give patients transparent information and refer them to support groups or psychologists if necessary.

6. Long-term follow-up :
Neuro-oncology patients require regular follow-up to monitor for signs of tumour recurrence, assess any long-term side-effects of treatment and adapt management.

7. Preparing for the trip :
Before leaving hospital, patients and their families need to be well informed about home care, medicines to take, warning signs to look out for and follow-up appointments.

8. Communication with a multidisciplinary team :
Collaboration between neurosurgeons, oncologists, radiologists, nurses, physiotherapists and other professionals is essential for comprehensive patient care.

The post-operative management of neuro-oncology patients is a multi-dimensional task that requires a holistic approach. The focus must be on medical monitoring, rehabilitation, emotional support and preparation for life after hospitalisation. Transparent communication and close coordination between the various healthcare professionals are essential to ensure the best possible outcome for the patient.

The role of the nurse in the overall care of the neuro-oncological patient

Nurses play a key role in the care of neuro-oncology patients, often being the closest link with patients and their families. Their strategic position between the medical team and the patient enables them to provide holistic care, ranging from medical care to emotional support.

1. Initial and ongoing assessment :
On admission, the nurse assesses the patient's state of health, history, symptoms and specific needs. This assessment is regularly updated to adapt care.

2. Treatment administration and monitoring :
Whether it's surgery, chemotherapy, radiotherapy or any other form of treatment, the nurse ensures that they are administered correctly and monitors any side effects or potential complications.

3. Education and advice :
The nurse informs the patient and his or her family about the disease, treatment and possible side-effects, as well as the preventive and self-care measures to be adopted.

4. Pain management :
The nurse regularly assesses the patient's pain, administers the appropriate analgesics and suggests non-pharmacological methods of relieving it.

5. Psychological support :
Faced with the shock of diagnosis and the challenges of treatment, nurses provide emotional support to patients and their families, and refer them to specialists if necessary.

6. Working with the multidisciplinary team :
Nurses work closely with neurosurgeons, oncologists, radiologists, physiotherapists and other health professionals to ensure coherent and comprehensive care.

7. Preparing for the trip :
The nurse ensures that the patient and their family are ready to manage the rest of their care at home, by providing information, advice and resources.

8. Long-term follow-up :
Even after discharge, the nurse can play a role in monitoring the patient, ensuring continuity of care, answering questions and facilitating follow-up appointments.

9. Research and continuing education :
Nurses keep abreast of the latest advances in neuro-oncology to provide the best possible care.

10. Prevention and health promotion :
Nurses can also play a role in raising awareness of brain tumour prevention, particularly in terms of risk factors and early signs.

Comprehensive care for neuro-oncology patients is a complex and multidimensional task. Nurses, through their proximity to patients, their expertise and their ability to work as part of a team, are key players in guaranteeing the quality and safety of care, while ensuring the well-being and emotional support of patients and their families.

Chapter 22:
THE IMPORTANCE OF NUTRITION IN NEUROSURGERY

Pre- and post-operative nutrition

Nutrition plays a vital role in the recovery of the neurosurgical patient. Adequate nutrition can accelerate healing, improve immune defences and contribute to a better convalescence. It requires particular attention, both before and after the operation.

Preoperative nutrition :

1. Metabolic preparation :
Before the operation, it is crucial to ensure that the patient is in an optimal nutritional state to better cope with the operation and its metabolic consequences. This may require dietary supplements rich in protein or other nutrients.

2. Hydration :
Maintaining adequate hydration is essential to avoid complications linked to dehydration, which could influence the dynamics of cerebrospinal fluid.

3. Preoperative food restriction :
Most patients are fasted before surgery to prevent the risk of aspiration during anaesthesia.

4. Glucose and electrolyte balance :
Ensure that glucose and electrolyte levels are within a normal range to avoid any intraoperative complications.

Postoperative nutrition :
1. Gradual reintroduction of food :
Depending on the type of surgery and the patient's condition, food is often gradually reintroduced, starting with clear liquids, then soft foods, and finally a normal diet.

2. Nutritional support :
Patients who are unable to eat orally may require enteral (tube) or parenteral (intravenous) feeding.

3. Symptom management :
Nausea, vomiting, constipation and other gastrointestinal complaints are common after surgery. Appropriate management may involve dietary changes, medication or other interventions.

4. Specific nutritional requirements :
After surgery, protein requirements are often increased to support tissue repair. In addition, increased requirements for vitamins and minerals, such as vitamin C and zinc, may be necessary for healing.

5. Hydration :
Hydration continues to be crucial after surgery to support renal function, healing and overall fluid balance.

6. Nutritional monitoring :
Regular assessment of the patient's nutritional status is essential to identify and rapidly treat any deficiencies or complications.

Nutritional management before and after neurosurgery is essential to optimise surgical results and speed recovery. It requires close collaboration between nurses, doctors, dieticians and other healthcare professionals to meet the specific needs of each patient.

Specific nutritional challenges neurosurgical patients

The nutritional management of neurosurgical patients is fraught with unique challenges, reflecting the complexity of the nervous system and its interactions with the rest of the body. These challenges are at the crossroads of the impact of the disease, the surgery itself and the specificities of neurological nutrition.

1. Dysphagia :

Many neurosurgical patients, particularly those who have undergone surgery to the brain stem or certain areas of the brain, may have difficulty swallowing. This makes swallowing solid food dangerous, as it can lead to a false route.

2. Impaired consciousness :

A reduced level of consciousness or cognitive fluctuations may complicate the patient's ability to eat independently. They may not recognise food or refuse to eat.

3. Metabolic changes :

Following brain injury or surgery, metabolism can be altered, increasing the patient's calorie and protein requirements.

4. Water restrictions :

Some patients may require fluid restrictions to manage cerebral oedema or other complications, making the management of nutrition and hydration tricky.

5. Increased risk of malnutrition :

The combination of anorexia, nausea, vomiting and other gastrointestinal symptoms can quickly lead to malnutrition, especially if these symptoms are not properly managed.

6. Drug interactions :

Neurosurgical patients are often on various medications that can affect appetite, nutrient absorption or cause gastrointestinal problems.

7. Electrolyte disturbances :

Electrolyte imbalances, such as hyponatremia, can occur after certain neurosurgical procedures, requiring strict monitoring and management of sodium intake.

8. Motor limitations :

Motor deficits or weaknesses can make it difficult for patients to feed themselves or use utensils.

9. Gastrointestinal problems :

Constipation is common, particularly in immobile patients or those on certain medications. It must be actively managed to ensure patient comfort and avoid complications.

10. Special nutritional requirements :
Certain conditions, such as epilepsy, may require specific diets, such as the ketogenic diet.

The nutritional challenges faced by neurosurgical patients require a multidisciplinary approach. The nurse plays an essential role in assessing nutritional status, monitoring food intake and tolerance, and collaborating with other healthcare professionals, such as dieticians and gastroenterologists, to ensure optimal nutritional management.

Working with nutritionists and dieticians

In the complex landscape of neurosurgery, collaboration between nurses and nutrition professionals is vital. Neurosurgical patients often have specific and complex nutritional needs, and achieving optimal nutritional management requires a synergy of skills.

1. Initial assessment :
On admission, the nurse will usually carry out an initial assessment of the patient, including their nutritional status. This assessment may include indicators such as weight, appetite, the presence of dysphagia or gastrointestinal disorders. If nutritional concerns are identified, the patient is usually referred to a nutritionist or dietician for further assessment.

2. Individualised nutrition plans :
Based on the initial assessment and the patient's specific needs, the dietician draws up a nutritional plan. The nurse, working closely with the dietician, plays an essential role in implementing this plan, ensuring that the patient receives the appropriate meals and monitoring their tolerance of these meals.

3. Education and advice :

Dieticians often provide specific advice and education on nutrition, while nurses reinforce this information in their day-to-day interactions with the patient. The two professionals work together to help the patient understand the importance of nutrition in their recovery and to encourage adherence to an appropriate diet.

4. Feeding tube management :

For patients who are unable to eat orally, enteral nutrition (via a tube) may be necessary. The nurse is generally responsible for administering this nutrition, while the dietician calculates the specific needs and formulates the enteral diet.

5. Continuous monitoring :

Nutritional needs may change over the course of a patient's convalescence. The nurse, in collaboration with the dietician, regularly monitors the patient's nutritional status, adjusting the care plan according to changing needs.

6. Interprofessional communication :

The success of nutritional management depends to a large extent on smooth, regular communication between the nurse and dietician. Multidisciplinary team meetings, shared medical notes and informal discussions are all tools that help to ensure effective collaboration.

Collaboration between nurses and nutrition professionals is essential to ensure the best possible care for neurosurgical patients. Each professional brings unique expertise, and by working together they can ensure that patients receive optimal nutrition, promoting faster recovery and better long-term outcomes.

Chapter 23:
THE PATIENT JOURNEY :
FROM DIAGNOSIS TO REHABILITATION

Detailed case studies to illustrate the complete patient journey

Case study 1: Mrs Dupont, aged 56 - Brain tumour
Initial presentation:
Mrs Dupont presented to hospital with persistent headaches, dizziness and impaired vision for several months. A brain MRI revealed a tumour in the right frontal lobe.

Pre-operative assessment and full work-up:
Full neurological tests are carried out, including cognitive function, vision and motor function tests. Blood work is normal. The neurosurgery team discusses the case with Mrs Dupont and the surgical option.

Psychological preparation:
A psychologist meets with Mrs Dupont to discuss her fears about surgery and offers emotional support.

Pre-operative phase:
The nurse prepares Mrs Dupont for surgery, explains the procedure, checks current medication and discusses post-operative care.

Intervention:
Mrs Dupont undergoes a craniotomy to remove the tumour. The operation went well, and the tumour was completely removed.

Post-operative care:
The nurse monitors Mrs Dupont's vital signs, pain, neurological signs and makes sure the patient is conscious and oriented.

Pain management :
Mrs Dupont receives analgesics and her pain level is regularly assessed.

Rehabilitation:
Once stable, Mrs Dupont is transferred to a rehabilitation unit where she works with physiotherapists, occupational therapists and other professionals to regain her strength and cognitive abilities.

Follow-up:
Mrs Dupont returns for regular post-operative check-ups, follow-up MRI scans and consultations with her neurosurgeon and oncologist.

Conclusion:
A few months after the operation, Mrs Dupont is feeling well, has resumed her daily activities and shows no signs of tumour recurrence.

Case study 2: Mr Bernard, aged 32 - Herniated disc
Initial presentation:
Mr Bernard complained of severe back pain radiating down his right leg. An MRI of the spine revealed a herniated L4-L5 disc.

Preoperative assessment and full work-up:
Physical examination confirms weakness of the right foot. Medical history, including medication, is assessed.

Psychological preparation:
Mr Bernard expresses concerns about the operation and receives psychological support.

Pre-operative phase:
The nurse prepares Mr Bernard for the operation, explaining the discectomy surgery that will be performed.
Intervention:
Mr Bernard underwent a microscopic discectomy, where the herniated disc fragment was removed.

Post-operative care:
The nurse monitors vital signs, pain and neurological function.

Pain management:
Mr Bernard receives medication to manage post-operative pain.

Patient education:
Before discharge, Mr Bernard is given instructions on activities to avoid, how to move properly and signs to look out for.

Follow-up:
Mr Bernard returned for post-operative consultations, and his follow-up showed a significant improvement in pain and neurological function.

Conclusion:
After a few weeks of rehabilitation, Mr Bernard returned to work and daily activities with no residual pain.

Multidisciplinary involvement : nurse, surgeon, physiotherapist, etc.

When treating patients requiring neurosurgical intervention, a multidisciplinary approach is essential to ensure holistic and comprehensive care. Neurosurgical patients face not just surgical issues, but a range of complex needs before, during and after surgery that require the involvement of a variety of professionals.

- **The surgeon: The** surgeon is obviously the mainstay of any neurosurgical operation. He assesses the need for surgery, plans and carries it out, and then manages the post-operative period. He is responsible for the overall therapeutic strategy.
- **The nurse:** Nurses play a key role throughout the patient's journey. They provide preoperative care, assist during surgery, and are essential in the postoperative phase to monitor the patient, administer medication, educate the patient and family, and coordinate with other professionals.
- **The physiotherapist:** After surgery, many patients require rehabilitation to restore motor function or manage pain. Physiotherapists help with early mobilisation, restoring function and teaching appropriate movement techniques.
- **The psychologist/psychiatrist:** Surgery, particularly neurosurgery, can be stressful for patients. Some may find it difficult to accept their diagnosis or cope with post-operative stress. Psychological support is crucial for these patients.
- **The nutritionist:** Good nutrition is essential for recovery. A nutritionist can assess a patient's specific dietary needs, suggest dietary modifications and help set up a diet for optimal recovery.
- **Occupational therapists: While** physiotherapists focus on motor function, occupational therapists help patients regain their independence in everyday activities, by adapting their environment or teaching new skills.
- **The social worker:** They can help coordinate home care, provide emotional support and help resolve any social or financial problems that may arise.

- **Other specialists:** Depending on the case, other specialists such as neurologists, radiologists, anaesthetists, oncologists, etc. may be involved in the treatment.

The collaboration between all these professionals ensures comprehensive care, from initial assessment through to long-term rehabilitation. This integrated approach ensures that patients receive not only high-quality medical care, but also emotional, social and physical support throughout their treatment. It is this combination that ultimately leads to optimal outcomes for the patient.

Discharge planning and follow-up care

Discharge planning is an essential stage in the care of a neurosurgical patient. It begins well in advance of the actual discharge date and involves meticulous coordination between various members of the medical team, the patient and his or her family. The aim is to ensure a smooth transition from hospital to home or another care facility, making sure that the patient has all the tools and support needed for optimal recovery.

- **Initial assessment:** Even before surgery, the medical team assesses the patient's potential needs after discharge. This may include specific needs in terms of rehabilitation, medication, equipment or home support.
- **Discussion with the patient and family:** It is essential to actively involve the patient and family in the planning. They need to understand the nature of post-operative care, the potential challenges and their responsibilities.
- **Coordination with healthcare professionals:** Discharge from hospital does not mean the end of

care. Home nurses, physiotherapists, occupational therapists and others may be needed to ensure continuity of care. Follow-up appointments with the surgeon and other specialists are also scheduled.

- **Preparing the home:** Depending on the nature of the surgery and the patient's condition, adaptations to the home may be necessary. This may include the installation of specific equipment, such as grab bars, ramps or healthcare beds.
- **Education and training:** Before discharge, patients and their families must be trained in home care, medication management, recognising the signs of complications and what to do in an emergency.
- **Medication plan:** A detailed medication plan, including dosage, frequency, potential side effects and interactions, is drawn up and shared with the patient.
- **Documentation:** All relevant details of the patient's hospital stay, surgery, post-operative care and follow-up recommendations are recorded in a document given to the patient.
- **Follow-up care:** Care does not stop at discharge. Follow-up appointments are used to monitor the patient's progress, identify and manage any complications and adjust care plans as necessary.
- **Emotional and psychological support:** The postoperative period can be emotionally trying. Psychological support services and support groups can be beneficial.
- **Discharge assessment:** A few weeks after discharge, it is useful to carry out an assessment to determine whether the patient's needs are being met and whether there are areas for improvement in future planning.

The key to a successful discharge and recovery lies in careful planning, transparent communication and close collaboration between all those involved.

Chapter 24:
FUTURE INNOVATIONS
IN NEUROSURGERY

A look at potential developments neurosurgery:
techniques, tools, approaches

Neurosurgery, the medical speciality dedicated to surgical interventions on the nervous system, has continued to evolve over the decades. While the twentieth century saw the birth and consolidation of basic surgical techniques, the twenty-first century is witnessing an explosion of innovative technologies and multidisciplinary approaches. Let's take a look at the current and future trends that could reshape this specialty.

- **Robotics in neurosurgery:** The use of robots in the operating theatre is no longer science fiction. These machines, piloted by surgeons, can perform operations with incredible precision, potentially reducing risks and improving outcomes for patients.
- **Artificial intelligence (AI):** With the advent of AI, neurosurgery could benefit from tools to aid diagnosis, surgical planning and even early warning systems for post-operative complications.
- **Image-guided surgery:** The fusion of images from different modalities (MRI, CT, ultrasound) during the operation enables the surgeon to 'see' beyond the apparent anatomical structures, offering greater precision.
- **Gene and cell therapies:** Rather than focusing solely on mechanical surgery, neurosurgery could incorporate gene or cell therapies to treat diseases

such as Parkinson's, brain tumours and other neurological conditions.

- **Less invasive techniques:** Neuroendoscopy, stereotactic surgery and endovascular techniques will continue to develop, offering procedures with smaller incisions, less bleeding and shorter recovery times.
- **3D bioprinting:** 3D printing of biological structures could one day make it possible to 'reconstruct' damaged areas of the brain or spinal cord.
- **Functional neurosurgery:** Techniques such as deep brain stimulation make it possible to treat neurological disorders without physically removing or altering brain tissue.
- **Telemedicine:** In an increasingly connected world, telemedicine will play a crucial role, not only for post-operative follow-up, but also for collaboration between specialists across the globe.
- **Training and simulation:** Neurosurgeon training programmes could make greater use of virtual reality and simulators to train future surgeons without risk to patients.
- **Multidisciplinary approach:** Collaboration between neurosurgeons, neurologists, radiologists and other specialists will be essential to tackle the complex challenges of the nervous system in a holistic way.

The future of neurosurgery looks bright, with a host of new techniques and tools that promise to improve patient outcomes while reducing the risks associated with surgery. These advances reflect the dynamic and innovative nature of modern medicine.

The influence of artificial intelligence and robotics

Over the years, artificial intelligence (AI) and robotics have become exponentially integrated into the medical field, bringing about major revolutions, particularly in the speciality of neurosurgery. Here's how these two transformative technologies have influenced and continue to influence this field of expertise.

1. Greater surgical precision :
Robots, controlled by surgeons, can perform operations with micrometric precision. In neurosurgery, where every millimetre counts, this means less damage to surrounding healthy tissue and significant improvements in patient outcomes.

2. Preoperative planning with AI :
AI-based systems can rapidly analyse medical imaging datasets to identify regions of interest, plan optimal trajectories and even predict potential outcomes based on different surgical strategies.

3. Simulations and training :
Virtual reality coupled with AI offers simulation environments for surgeons in training. These simulators can reproduce complex scenarios, enabling surgeons to train without risk to real patients.

4. Real-time assistance :
During procedures, AI can provide real-time information, help with navigation and offer predictive analyses, for example, to anticipate bleeding or other complications.

5. Postoperative improvements :
AI systems can monitor a patient's vital signs and other data to quickly identify signs of complications, speeding up medical intervention in the event of a problem.

6. Telemedicine :
With the advent of digital platforms, surgeons can consult colleagues around the world, seek second opinions or even guide procedures remotely, all facilitated by AI systems.

7. Personalised care :
AI can help analyse large and complex datasets to provide personalised information about each patient, enabling more targeted and effective care.

8. Automation of routine tasks :
Many tasks, such as taking images or monitoring vital signs, can be automated using robotics, allowing medical staff to concentrate on more crucial aspects of care.

9. Flexible robotics :
The latest advances in robotics include flexible instruments that can adapt to the complex anatomy of the brain, providing access to areas that were previously difficult to reach.

10. Research and development :
AI can rapidly analyse huge databases to aid research, whether to identify trends, correlations or even to help design new surgical techniques.

The combined influence of artificial intelligence and robotics in neurosurgery has not only improved standards of care but also opened the door to new possibilities that were unimaginable just a few decades ago. These advances, while posing new ethical and technical challenges, promise a bright future for the specialty and, above all, for the patients it serves.

Preparing and adapting nurses to these changes

Faced with rapid advances in neurosurgery, specifically with the introduction of artificial intelligence and robotics, nurses, as essential links in the care chain, must adapt and prepare themselves to remain relevant and effective. Here's how:

1. Continuing education :
It is crucial for nurses to attend regular training courses to keep up to date with the latest techniques and technologies. This may include courses, workshops or seminars on robotics, AI or other relevant innovations.

2. Simulations and practical training :
Like surgeons, nurses can benefit from simulations to familiarise themselves with new technologies without risk to patients. This allows them to practise their skills in a controlled environment.

3. Multidisciplinary collaboration :
Nurses need to work closely with surgeons, technicians and other professionals to understand and adapt to changes. Regular communication and teamwork are essential.

4. Updating protocols :
With the introduction of new technologies, care protocols may need to be revised. Nurses need to be proactive in reviewing and adapting these protocols to ensure safe and effective care.

5. Flexibility and open-mindedness :
The medical landscape is changing rapidly. Open-mindedness and a willingness to embrace change, however daunting it may be at first, are crucial to adaptation.

6. Ethics and sensitivity :
The introduction of new technologies often raises new ethical questions. Nurses need to be trained to recognise and navigate these dilemmas, while always putting the patient's well-being first.

7. Computer skills :
With the rise of technology, having a basic understanding of computer systems and medical software has become almost as important as mastering traditional clinical skills.

8. Participation in research :
Nurses can play an active role in clinical research, helping to assess the effectiveness and safety of new technologies while sharing their unique perspectives.

9. Patient empowerment :
With increased access to information, patients are more informed than ever. Nurses can play a crucial role in educating patients about new technologies, dispelling myths and concerns.

10. Preventing burnout :
Constant adaptation to new technologies can be stressful. So it's vital that nurses recognise the signs of burnout and adopt prevention strategies.

In this world of rapid technological progress, nurses remain a pillar of humanity, ethics and patient-centred care. By embracing change while preserving these core values, nurses will continue to provide exceptional care despite the changing medical landscape.

Chapter 25:
CONTINUITY OF CARE
AND RETURN HOME

Discharge planning and coordination with home care

Discharge planning for neurosurgical patients and coordination with home care are essential steps in ensuring a smooth transition from hospital to home and continuity of care. This transition is critical to avoiding unnecessary re-hospitalisation, managing symptoms effectively and improving the patient's quality of life. Here's how this process can be orchestrated successfully:

1. Overall assessment of the patient :
Before discharge, a full assessment is carried out to determine the level of care required, equipment needs, medication required and other health considerations.

2. Patient and family education :
Clear information on post-operative management, medication, warning signs and follow-up procedures is shared with the patient and their family. This gives them the tools they need to manage the situation at home.

3. Coordination with home care :
Depending on the patient's needs, a homecare team can be put in place, including nurses, physiotherapists, occupational therapists, etc. Their integration is planned before discharge to ensure a smooth transition. Their integration is planned before discharge to ensure a smooth transition.

4. Medical prescription and follow-up :
A clear medication plan is drawn up, with coordination to ensure that prescriptions are filled and accessible. Follow-up appointments are also scheduled with the neurosurgeon or other specialists.

5. Home equipment and modifications :
Depending on the patient's needs, specific equipment (such as healthcare beds, wheelchairs, etc.) may be required. Home modifications may also be recommended to facilitate mobility and safety.

6. Emotional and psychological support :
Recognise that discharge, although a positive step, can also be a source of anxiety for patients and their families. Psychological resources or support groups may be suggested.

7. Open communication lines :
It is essential to establish clear lines of communication between the patient, the family, the homecare providers and the medical team. This enables any concerns or problems that may arise to be dealt with quickly.

8. Regular reassessments :
Follow-up home visits or teleconsultations can be scheduled to assess the patient's progress and adjust care if necessary.

9. Involvement of carers :
Carers play a crucial role in home care. They need to be involved in the planning process, receive appropriate training and ongoing support.

10. Full documentation :
All details of the patient's care, interventions and recommendations must be fully documented to ensure continuity of care.

Discharge planning and coordination with home care requires a holistic, patient-centred approach, where every detail is taken into account to ensure the patient's well-being and safety.

Ensuring a smooth transition for the patient

The transition from hospital to home is a major stage in a patient's care, particularly after neurosurgery. This period can be marked by uncertainty and anxiety, but also by the hope of recovery and an improved life. A smooth transition is therefore essential for the patient's well-being and to minimise post-operative risks. Here's how it can be done:

1. Continuing education :
Before discharge, it is essential to provide the patient and family with detailed information about post-operative care, medication, activities to be avoided, and signs and symptoms requiring immediate medical attention. A clear understanding of what to expect can reduce anxiety and improve compliance.

2. Advance planning :
Preparations for discharge should begin well before the actual day of discharge. This includes coordinating with the home care teams, obtaining prescriptions and medical equipment, and setting up a medical monitoring plan.

3. Close monitoring :
The first few days after discharge are crucial. Organising home visits, follow-up calls or teleconsultations helps to ensure that everything is going well, to answer the patient's questions and to deal with any complications quickly.

4. Clear lines of communication :
Patients and their families need to know who to contact in the event of a problem. Providing emergency contact numbers, as well as a list of signs and symptoms that require medical intervention, is essential.

5. Psychological support :
The transition can be emotionally challenging. Offering psychological support, whether through individual consultations or support groups, is a key step in ensuring the patient's mental well-being.

6. Integration of carers :
Relatives who take on the role of carers need to be trained and supported. Their role is essential for a smooth transition. They should be equipped with the skills needed to help the patient and be aware of the resources available if necessary.

7. Rehabilitation and physiotherapy :
If necessary, rehabilitation or physiotherapy sessions can be organised at home or in a specialist centre to help patients regain their independence.
8. Pain management :
Effective management of postoperative pain is essential for patient comfort and recovery. This requires good communication between the patient, their carers and the medical team.

9. Social reintegration :
Encouraging patients to gradually resume their social activities and hobbies can make a major contribution to their emotional and physical recovery.

Ensuring a smooth transition for the patient requires a multidisciplinary, patient-centred approach. With careful planning, open communication and ongoing support, the patient is more likely to experience this transition as a positive step towards healing and recovery.

Educating patients and their families on post-operative care

After neurosurgery, postoperative education for the patient and family is crucial. A good understanding of the care required and potential complications can reduce anxiety, speed up recovery and prevent future problems.

1. Clear explanation of the procedure :
It is essential to review what has been achieved during the operation, so that the patient and his or her family fully understand the post-operative implications and expectations.

2. Wound care :
Detailed instructions should be provided on how to clean and care for any surgical incision, including signs of infection or other complications to look out for.

3. Physical activities :
The patient should be informed of the activities to be avoided, the need for rest and the gradual resumption of movement and exercise.

4. Medication :
A list of prescribed medicines, their dosages, frequency and possible side effects should be provided. It is also important to stress the importance of adhering to the medication regime.

5. Nutrition and hydration :
Depending on the procedure, specific guidelines for feeding and fluid intake may be necessary. These must be clearly explained.

6. Warning signs :
Report any symptoms requiring immediate medical attention, such as high fever, severe headaches, blurred vision or speech, weakness or numbness, etc.

7. Medical follow-up :
Inform patients and their families about follow-up appointments, their frequency and their importance in monitoring progress and identifying any complications early on.

8. Emotional support :
Surgery, especially neurosurgery, can have an emotional impact. It is important to discuss any postoperative mood or sleep problems and to suggest resources or professionals who can help.

9. Resources available :
Provide a list of resources, such as emergency telephone numbers, patient associations or support groups.

10. Involvement of carers :
Educate those who will be most closely involved with the patient, giving them clear guidelines and reassuring them of their essential role in the recovery process.

11. Rehabilitation :
If necessary, talk about the rehabilitation and physiotherapy options available and their importance for a full recovery.

Postoperative education is a collaborative process. It is vital to encourage patients and their families to ask questions and express their concerns. By providing clear and comprehensive information, offering support and establishing open communication, the healing process can be greatly facilitated.

Chapter 26:
CAREER MANAGEMENT AND PROFESSIONAL DEVELOPMENT

Continuing training opportunities and specialisation

Neurosurgery is a constantly evolving field. With the emergence of new technologies, techniques and knowledge, nurses working in neurosurgery must continually update their skills. Continuing education and specialisation are essential to providing the highest quality care and staying at the cutting edge.

1. Courses and workshops :
Many hospitals, professional associations and institutions offer courses and workshops focusing on advances in neurosurgery, patient management, new technologies and many other relevant topics.

2. Advanced diplomas :
For those who wish to deepen their knowledge, there are master's or doctoral programmes in nursing with a concentration in neuroscience or surgical care.

3. Certifications :
Obtaining certification in a specific field, such as neurosurgical or critical care, can not only improve skills but also professional credibility. Many organisations offer certifications that require hours of training, practical experience and passing an exam.

4. Seminars and conferences :
Attending national or international conferences not only allows you to learn about the latest developments in the field, but also to network with other professionals and exchange experiences and ideas.

5. Publications and research :
Reading professional journals, participating in research or even publishing your own findings or case studies can enrich knowledge and contribute to the advancement of the field.

6. Online training :
With the rise of technology, many courses and training are now available online, offering flexibility and convenience.

7. Additional specialisations :
Depending on interest, a neurosurgery nurse may choose to specialise further in areas such as neuro-oncology, paediatric surgery, neurological rehabilitation, etc.

8. Teaching and mentoring :
Passing on your knowledge to the next generation of nurses or becoming a mentor for less experienced nurses can also be a way of learning and contributing to the profession.

9. Involvement in associations :
Joining professional associations specific to neurosurgery or nursing in general can offer training opportunities, resources, scholarships and a professional network.

10. Interdisciplinary collaboration :
Working closely with other healthcare professionals, such as neurosurgeons, radiologists and anaesthetists, can provide a unique perspective and deepen understanding of holistic care.

Continuous learning is not only beneficial to a nurse's career, it is also essential to ensure that patients receive the safest, most effective and up-to-date care possible. In the fast-paced and complex world of neurosurgery, a commitment to continuous learning is essential.

Managing balance work-life in neurosurgery

The field of neurosurgery is demanding, both physically and emotionally. Professionals in this speciality, whether surgeons, nurses or other members of the medical team, are often faced with tense situations, irregular working hours and unexpected emergencies. In this context, finding a balance between professional responsibilities and personal life is crucial to preventing burnout and maintaining good mental health.

1. Planning and organisation :
The key is to anticipate and plan ahead. Using a diary or a planning application to manage schedules, set rest periods and mark out times for leisure activities or family can help avoid overwork.

2. Prioritising mental and physical health :
It's essential to recognise your own limits. Incorporating activities such as sport, meditation or even creative hobbies can help to manage stress. In addition, consulting a mental health professional or counsellor can provide tools for managing the complex emotions associated with this profession.

3. Take regular holidays :
Although it may seem difficult to get away from work, a holiday or even a short break can help you recharge your batteries and prevent burnout.

4. Setting limits :
It's crucial to know how to say no when necessary and to define boundaries between work and home. Avoiding bringing work home and disconnecting from work emails or calls during free time can help maintain this balance.

5. Seek support :
Talking to colleagues or mentors who have managed to find a balance can offer useful insights and strategies. Support from family and friends can also help manage the pressures of work.

6. Flexibility :
If possible, negotiating flexible working hours or the possibility of working remotely can help to balance professional and personal responsibilities.

7. Further training :
Continuing education, not only in neurosurgery but also in time management, communication and well-being, can provide tools and skills to better manage balance.

8. Cultivating passions outside work :
Having activities or passions outside neurosurgery can provide an escape and a way of decompressing.

9. Reassess regularly :
Work-life balance is not static. It's essential to take the time to reflect regularly on your situation, assess what's working and what's not, and adjust accordingly.

10. Accept that perfection is not always possible:
There will be days when balance seems out of reach. At those times, it's important to remember that everyone is doing their best and that balance is an ongoing process.

Although neurosurgery is a demanding profession, it is possible to find a balance. It requires self-awareness, careful planning, and the support of a community, but the benefits of a balanced career are well worth the effort.

Professional network and participation conferences and symposia

The rapid development of medicine, and neurosurgery in particular, means that knowledge needs to be constantly updated. In this context, the importance of professional networking and participation in conferences and symposia is invaluable. They provide an opportunity not only for learning, but also for collaboration and exchange.

1. Benefits of professional networking :
   - **Exchanging expertise**: Networking enables professionals to share their experiences, research and discoveries, thereby enriching each other's practice.
   - **Opportunities for collaboration**: Meeting other experts in the field can open the door to new collaborations in research, publications or clinical projects.
   - **Career development**: The professional network can lead to job opportunities, mentoring offers or academic collaborations.
   - **Moral and emotional support**: Sharing challenges and successes with colleagues who understand the demanding nature of the job can provide essential psychological support.
2. The value of conferences and symposia :
   - **Updating knowledge**: These events are often an opportunity for experts to present the latest advances, surgical techniques or discoveries in neurosurgery.

- **Practical workshops**: Many symposia offer workshops where participants can get hands-on training in the latest techniques or technologies.
- **Presenting research**: Conferences are often a platform for presenting research work, receiving feedback and establishing a reputation in the field.
- **Interdisciplinary meetings**: These events often bring together experts from various related fields, encouraging an interdisciplinary approach to patient care.

3. Maximising the benefits of conferences :
- **Preparation**: Before taking part, it's a good idea to familiarise yourself with the agenda, choose the relevant sessions and prepare any questions or discussions.
- **Active participation**: Rather than simply being a spectator, active involvement, such as asking questions or taking part in debates, maximises the benefits of the event.
- **Networking**: Use breaks and social events to meet and talk to other participants.
- **Follow-up**: After the event, get in touch with the people you meet and explore possibilities for collaboration or exchange.

Professional networking and active participation in conferences and symposia are central to professional growth in neurosurgery. They promote continuous learning, collaboration and the advancement of the profession as a whole.

Chapter 27:
SAFETY AT WORK
AND RISK PREVENTION

Specific risks neurosurgery (radiation, ergonomics, etc.).

As a medical discipline, neurosurgery presents a range of specific risks for the professionals who work in it. These risks are intrinsic to the complexity of the operations, the technologies used, and the delicate nature of the nervous system. Here is an overview of the main risks faced by neurosurgeons and the medical team who work with them.

1. Exposure to radiation :
Many neurosurgical procedures require the use of real-time imaging, such as fluoroscopy, to guide the surgeon during the operation.
   • **Risks**: Repeated exposure to radiation can increase the risk of illnesses such as cancer, as well as other conditions.
   • **Prevention**: It is crucial to limit exposure time, use protective screens and wear protective clothing such as lead aprons.

2. Ergonomics and musculoskeletal disorders :
Surgeons spend many hours in a static position, often in non-ergonomic postures, bending over or turning their necks to get a better view of the operating field.
   • **Risks**: These postures can lead to chronic pain, musculoskeletal disorders and long-term injuries.
   • **Prevention**: Using ergonomic supports, taking regular breaks to stretch the body, and ergonomic training can help minimise these risks.

3. Infectious risks :
Despite a sterile environment, neurosurgery exposes both patients and medical staff to the risk of infection.
- **Risks**: Infections can be transmitted through blood or other body fluids.
- **Prevention**: It is essential to follow sterilisation protocols scrupulously, to use personal protective equipment and to keep up to date with best practice.

4. Fatigue and stress :
The demanding nature of neurosurgery, the long working hours and the crucial decisions to be made can lead to mental and physical fatigue.
- **Risks**: Fatigue can compromise concentration, increase the risk of error and affect mental health.
- **Prevention**: It's important to have a good work-life balance, take breaks and have the resources to manage stress.

5. Exposure to chemicals :
The use of disinfectants, sterilisation products and other chemical substances is common in neurosurgery.
- **Risks**: Exposure may cause allergic reactions, irritation or other health problems.
- **Prevention**: It is recommended to use appropriate personal protective equipment, to work in well-ventilated areas and to follow the recommendations on the use and disposal of products.

Although neurosurgery is an exciting and rewarding discipline, it also involves specific risks. Awareness of these risks and ongoing training in preventive best practice are essential to ensure the safety and well-being of healthcare professionals.

Preventive measures and good practice

Neurosurgery, with its delicate nature and potential implications for patients' quality of life, requires a meticulous approach to minimise risks. To ensure the safety of patients and healthcare professionals, certain preventive measures and good practices are essential. Here is a summary of the key measures to adopt:

1. Sterilisation and disinfection :
   - **Measures**: Ensure the sterility of surgical instruments and the operating field, use effective disinfecting agents and scrupulously follow sterilisation protocols.
   - **Good practice**: Regularly train staff in the latest sterilisation techniques and periodically check the efficiency of processes.
2. Protection against radiation :
   - **Measures**: Limit the time of exposure to radiation, use protective screens and wear protective equipment such as lead aprons when using imaging equipment.
   - **Good practice**: Educate staff about the dangers of radiation and ensure that imaging equipment is regularly maintained and calibrated.
3. Ergonomics in the operating theatre :
   - **Measures**: Invest in ergonomic equipment, such as adjustable tables and chairs, and encourage surgeons to adopt correct postures during surgery.
   - **Best practice**: Organise workshops on ergonomics and encourage staff to take breaks to stretch their bodies.
4. Infection prevention :
   - **Measures**: Use personal protective equipment, such as gloves, masks and gowns, and strictly follow hygiene protocols.

- **Good practice**: Provide ongoing training in hygiene techniques and regularly monitor hospital infection rates.

5. Managing stress and fatigue :
   - **Measures**: Encourage a healthy work-life balance, put in place psychological support systems for staff, and promote reasonable working hours.
   - **Best practice**: Organise awareness-raising sessions on stress management and offer wellness programmes.

6. Further training :
   - **Measures**: Promote ongoing training to keep staff up to date with the latest techniques, research and protocols in neurosurgery.
   - **Best practice**: Offer opportunities to participate in conferences, workshops and seminars, and encourage the exchange of experience between professionals.

7. Review of incidents :
   - **Measures**: Set up an incident reporting system to analyse and learn from errors or complications.
   - **Best practice**: Organise review meetings to discuss incidents in a non-judgmental way, in order to understand the root causes and prevent recurrence.

By adopting these preventive measures and good practices, neurosurgery can continue to progress while ensuring the safety of the patients and professionals involved.

Intervention protocols in the event of an incident

In neurosurgery, given the delicacy and complexity of the discipline, the establishment of incident response protocols is crucial to ensure the safety and well-being of patients. Here is an outline of the general steps that could be included in such a protocol:

1. Initial assessment :
   - **Identify the nature and seriousness of the incident**: is it a haemorrhage, unintentional nerve damage, an equipment problem or something else?
   - **Stabilising the patient**: Ensuring that the patient's vital functions are stable, including breathing, circulation and level of consciousness.
2. Communication :
   - **Inform the team**: Ensure that all members of the surgical team are aware of the incident and the corrective measures underway.
   - **Notify the department manager or supervisor**: This is where you can get additional assistance or advice on how to manage the incident.
3. Immediate intervention :
   - **Stop the source of the problem**: For example, in the case of bleeding, try to control the haemorrhage.
   - **Repair the injury**: If possible, immediately repair any injury or damage caused.
   - **Document the incident**: It is crucial to document precisely what happened, the measures taken and any changes in the patient's condition.
4. Post-incident management :
   - **Monitoring the patient**: Close monitoring of the patient is essential to detect any complications or side effects resulting from the incident.
   - **Informing the family**: The patient's family must be kept informed, as far as possible, in an honest and transparent manner.
   - **Analysis of the incident**: It is important to understand the root cause of the incident to avoid recurrences.

5. Evaluation and improvement :
 - **Debriefing meetings**: Bring the team together to discuss the incident, identify lessons learned and define measures to prevent it happening again.
 - **Updating protocols**: Depending on the nature of the incident, it may be necessary to review and adjust current protocols.
 - **Training and awareness**: Organise training sessions to reinforce good practice and prevent future incidents.
6. Support :
 - **Psychological support for the team**: Incidents can have an emotional impact on the team. It is important to offer them psychological support if necessary.
 - **Support for the patient and their family**: They may need psychological support or additional information to deal with the consequences of the incident.

It is important to stress that these general steps must be adapted specifically to each institution and each type of incident. Preparation, ongoing training and regular review of protocols are essential to ensure an effective response to neurosurgical incidents.

Chapter 28:
CONTINUING EDUCATION
AND FUTURE PROSPECTS

Importance of updating
skills and knowledge

Constantly updating skills and knowledge is fundamental in the medical field, and particularly in neurosurgery, a discipline that is evolving rapidly with the emergence of new techniques, technologies and research. Here are just a few of the reasons why this is so important:

- **Rapidly evolving technology and techniques:** Medical technology, particularly in the field of neurosurgery, is evolving at breakneck speed. New equipment, new methods of intervention and less invasive procedures are constantly being developed. To provide the best possible care, healthcare professionals need to be at the cutting edge of these innovations.
- **Improving patient safety:** Up-to-date knowledge helps to avoid medical errors, better anticipate possible complications and apply best practice to ensure patient safety.
- **Increased efficiency of care:** Up-to-date skills can reduce recovery time, minimise post-operative pain and improve long-term outcomes for patients.
- **Professional standards and regulations :** Medical regulatory bodies often set standards that require continuing education. Failure to comply with these standards may have legal or professional consequences.

- **Professional competition:** In a competitive medical world, keeping abreast of the latest advances can be a definite advantage, whether in terms of peer recognition, career progression or attracting patients.
- **Patient confidence:** Patients are increasingly well informed thanks to access to information via the internet. An up-to-date professional increases patients' confidence in their abilities and in the quality of the care they receive.
- **Intellectual stimulation and job satisfaction:** Continuous learning can be a source of motivation, enabling professionals to remain passionate and committed to their work.
- **Interdisciplinary collaboration:** As knowledge evolves, the boundaries between different medical specialities can sometimes become blurred. Regular updates help to improve collaboration and mutual understanding between specialities.
- **Preventing burnout:** Feeling stagnant or overwhelmed can contribute to burnout. Continuing training can offer renewal, a new perspective and a sense of accomplishment.
- **Professional ethics: Ultimately, it is the** ethical responsibility of every healthcare professional to ensure that he or she provides the best possible care. This can only be achieved through a commitment to continuous learning.

So updating skills and knowledge is not just desirable; it is imperative. It ensures that healthcare professionals can deliver the highest quality care, adapt to the changing challenges of the medical field and maintain a fulfilling and successful career.

Technological advances and their impact on nursing practice in neurosurgery

Technological advances have revolutionised the world of medicine, and neurosurgery in particular. This has inevitably had a profound impact on nursing practice. Here is an exploration of that impact:

- **Advanced medical imaging:** The introduction of cutting-edge imaging technologies such as functional MRI, tractography and neuronavigation has enabled more precise visualisation of the brain. For nurses, this means better pre-operative preparation, more precise monitoring during the operation and improved post-operative assessment.
- **Robotics and computer assistance:** Computer-guided surgical robots offer unrivalled precision in certain operations. Nurses now need to work closely with these technologies, ensure they function properly and be trained in their use.
- **Telemedicine:** Digital platforms now enable remote patient monitoring, virtual consultations and online follow-up. This has changed the way nurses interact with patients and other healthcare professionals.
- **Applications and connected objects:** Smartwatches, symptom-tracking applications and other devices can help monitor patients' neurological condition. Nurses need to be trained in how to use these tools, how to integrate them into the care plan, and how to interpret the data.
- **Electronic patient record management systems:** These systems enable better coordination of care, more accurate documentation and faster access to crucial information. Nurses now need to be comfortable with these technologies.

- **Virtual reality training:** Virtual reality now offers immersive training platforms, enabling nurses to practise managing complex situations in a controlled environment.
- **3D printing:** Used to create models of the brain or spine, 3D printing can help medical teams plan complex interventions. Nurses can use these models to explain procedures to patients or to prepare for specific interventions.
- **New medical devices:** Technological advances have led to the introduction of more sophisticated medical devices for monitoring and treatment. Nurses need to be trained in their use, maintenance and rapid detection of malfunctions.
- **Biomarkers and genomics:** Advances in research into biomarkers and genomics could lead to personalised care for patients. Nurses will need to understand these concepts and their implications for treatment.
- **Advanced alert systems:** Integrated devices can now detect changes in a patient's condition at an early stage and alert carers. Nurses need to be responsive to these alerts and act accordingly.

The impact of technological advances on neurosurgical nursing practice is profound. They offer invaluable tools for improving patient care, but also require ongoing training, adaptability and regular updating of skills. While these innovations are promising, they also place greater responsibility on nurses to ensure that they are used to best effect in the service of patients.

Building a rewarding career: specialisations and opportunities growth

Building a rewarding career in the medical field, and for nurses in particular, requires both a long-term vision and adaptability to the constant changes in the healthcare sector. Here's how you can structure your career, focusing on specialisations and growth opportunities:

1. Basic education and initial training :
   - It all starts with solid initial training. Obtaining a nursing diploma is the first step, but the journey doesn't end there.
   - Clinical placements during training are essential for understanding where the future nurse's passion lies, whether in paediatrics, intensive care, neurosurgery or any other field.
2. First job and clinical experience :
   - The first few years of practice are crucial. They allow you to gain practical experience, familiarise yourself with the pace of work and understand the nuances of the nursing role.
   - It is essential to remain open to learning, to seek advice from more experienced colleagues and to take part in ongoing training.
3. Specialisations :
   - Once nurses have gained some experience, they may consider specialising in a particular area. This may include specialisations such as nurse anaesthetist, nurse practitioner, or intensive care nurse, to name but a few.
   - Obtaining certification in a specialty can improve job prospects, increase earning potential and offer opportunities in cutting-edge areas of medicine.

4. Advanced education :
   - Obtaining a postgraduate degree, such as a master's or doctorate in nursing, can open many doors. It can lead to roles in leadership, education, research or advanced practice.
   - This stage can also be a stepping stone into related fields, such as hospital administration, health policy or public health.
5. Leadership roles :
   - With experience and education comes the opportunity to take on leadership roles. These roles may include managing a team of nurses, overseeing the operations of a unit or department, or even running a healthcare facility.
   - Leadership skills can be enhanced through specific training, seminars and workshops.
6. Professional involvement :
   - Participating in professional organisations, attending conferences, publishing articles and carrying out research are all ways of keeping abreast of the latest developments and expanding your professional network.
   - It can also lead to consulting, teaching or public speaking opportunities.
7. Mentoring :
   - After gaining significant experience, becoming a mentor for young nurses can be very rewarding. Passing on your knowledge and helping others to grow is a valuable way of giving back to the profession.
8. Work-life balance :
   - As your career develops, it's essential to keep an eye on the balance between work and personal life. Taking care of your mental and physical health, spending time with family and friends, and pursuing passions outside of work are crucial to a sustainable and rewarding career.

9. Preparing for retirement :
- As the end of your career approaches, it's wise to start planning for retirement. This can include financial considerations, but also thinking about how you want to spend your time in retirement, whether that's travelling, volunteering or pursuing other passions.

Building a rewarding career as a nurse requires planning, continuous education, focused specialisation, and adaptability to the changes and challenges of the healthcare sector. Each stage offers its own rewards and challenges, and it's essential to take a long-term view while enjoying the journey at every stage.

Chapter 29:
CONCLUSIONS AND THOUGHTS

The neurosurgery nurse's obstacle course: passion, challenge and dedication

The journey of the neurosurgical nurse is an obstacle-filled one, requiring a combination of technical expertise, emotional resilience and sheer determination. This path, though arduous, is marked by a burning passion for medicine, an unshakeable will to overcome challenges and a deep devotion to patients.

Passion is the first fire that ignites these health professionals. From the very first days of their training, they are captivated by the complexity of the brain, that marvel of architecture that holds the secrets of consciousness, memory and personality. They are fascinated by neurosurgery's ability to intervene directly on this organ, to improve and even save lives. This passion is what drives them to immerse themselves in hours of study, practice and simulations, to keep abreast of technological advances and to constantly seek to perfect their skills.

The challenges, however, are constant. Each patient is a unique case, with his or her own history, fears and hopes. Nurses must not only master a range of technical skills, but also develop the emotional intelligence to manage the most stressful and uncertain moments. Complications can arise, decisions have to be taken quickly, and every action or inaction can have lasting consequences.

But it's the dedication to patients that lies at the heart of this profession. The neurosurgical nurse is not only the guarantor of patient safety during a procedure, they are also the reassuring face on awakening, the calming voice in moments of doubt, the unfailing support in the healing process. This dedication extends well beyond the operating theatre: it encompasses pre-operative consultations, post-operative care and long-term support.

The journey of the neurosurgical nurse is not just a career. It is a vocation, a mission. It is shaped by an unwavering passion for discovery and service, a determination to overcome every challenge encountered, and an unrivalled dedication to those entrusted to their care. In this delicate dance between science and humanity, the neurosurgical nurse emerges as an essential pillar, weaving together the threads of competence, compassion and courage.

Additional resources
to deepen your knowledge

To further your knowledge of neurosurgery, here are a few recommended resources that may be particularly useful for nurses and anyone else interested in the field:

- Books and manuals :
    - **"Greenberg's Handbook of Neurosurgery**: A comprehensive textbook covering a wide range of neurosurgical topics.
    - **"Neurology for the Non-Neurologist"**: A guide for those seeking to understand the basics of neurology and the surgical implications.
- Trade journals :
    - Journal of Neurosurgery (JNS)
    - Neurosurgery

- World Neurosurgery
- These journals contain research articles, case studies and other recent scientific contributions in the field.
- Associations and organisations :
  - World Federation of Neurosurgical Societies (WFNS)
  - American Association of Neurological Surgeons (AANS)
  - European Association of Neurosurgical Societies (EANS)
  - These associations offer resources, training, conferences and networking opportunities for professionals in the field.
- Online training and webinars :
  - **Coursera, Udemy, EdX**: Many universities and institutions offer free or paid online courses in neurology and neurosurgery.
  - **AANS Webinars**: For regular updates on advances and current practices.
- Digital applications and tools :
  - **Touch Surgery**: A surgical simulation application that allows users to practise and visualise surgical procedures.
  - **NeuroMind**: An application offering clinical scores, anatomical guides and other tools for neurosurgery professionals.
- Podcasts :
  - **Neurosurgery Podcast**: Covers a variety of topics related to neurosurgery, from discussions of the latest research to interviews with experts in the field.
- Forums and discussion groups :
  - **Neurosurgery Hub**: A forum where professionals can ask questions, share experiences and discuss the latest advances.

- Conferences and symposia :
- Attending specialist conferences is a great way to keep abreast of the latest research, talk to other professionals and take part in practical workshops.
- Research centres and specialist hospitals :
  - Visit or collaborate with renowned institutions such as the **Mayo Clinic**, **Johns Hopkins**, or other leading neurosurgical centres to deepen expertise.

Here is a list of relevant resources to help them learn more:
- Books and manuals :
  - **"Neurosurgery"** by Guillaume Lot and Emmanuel Mandonnet: An essential textbook for neurosurgery students and professionals.
  - **"Atlas of neurosurgery"**: A visual guide detailing common procedures and techniques.
- Trade journals :
  - **Neurosurgery**: The official journal of the French Society of Neurosurgery, publishing research articles, reviews and case studies.
  - **Journal de Neuroradiologie**: Focused on neuroradiology, but relevant to those in neurosurgery.
- Associations and organisations :
  - **Société Française de Neurochirurgie (SFNC):** The organisation offers resources, training, conferences and networking opportunities for professionals in the field in France.
  - **Association des Neurochirurgiens de Langue Française (ANLF):** Promotes exchanges between French-speaking neurosurgeons.
- Online training and webinars :
  - **Université Numérique Francophone Mondiale (UNFM):** offers free online courses

on various medical subjects, including neurosurgery.

- **SFNC Webinars**: Regular updates on current advances and best practice.
- Forums and discussion groups :
  - Some general medical forums, such as **Remede.org**, have sections dedicated to neurosurgery where professionals can exchange ideas.
- Conferences and symposia :
  - The SFNC and other similar organisations regularly organise specialist conferences and workshops in France and other French-speaking countries.

- Research centres and specialist hospitals :
  - Establishments such as the **Pitié-Salpêtrière** Hospital in Paris and the **Bordeaux University Hospital,** among others, are renowned centres for neurosurgery and often offer specialist training, workshops and research.
- Podcasts and media :
- While neurosurgery podcasts in French may be rarer, it's always a good idea to check platforms like Spotify or Apple Podcasts regularly for French-language medical programmes that might cover related topics.

It is always advisable to check the relevance and credibility of resources, especially when it comes to medical information. Participation in professional networks, associations or academic institutions can also help to identify and access the best resources available.

Inspiring the next generation
of dedicated nurses

Nursing is a unique blend of science, art, dedication and passion. At every turn in history, dedicated nurses have left an indelible mark, responding to the needs of the sick, supporting families in distress, and shaping healthcare policy around the world. Today, in the face of a rapidly changing society and unprecedented medical challenges, it is crucial to inspire the next generation of dedicated nurses.

Imagine a young adult, perhaps unsure of his or her path, but with an innate desire to help others. How do you show them the beauty, complexity and deep satisfaction that nursing can bring? It starts by telling stories, of patients whose lives have been transformed by the care and attention of a nurse, or of nurses themselves who have braved storms to provide vital care.

Educational institutions also have a vital role to play. They must not only equip students with the necessary technical skills, but also nurture that spark of empathy, that thirst to understand human beings in all their facets. Curricula must reflect the changing reality of the medical world while preserving the humanistic essence of the profession.

It is also important to break down stereotypes. Nurses are not just auxiliary figures in the shadow of doctors. They are health professionals in their own right, capable of clinical judgment, research and innovation. Let's highlight examples of nursing leaders, researchers and entrepreneurs who are pushing the boundaries of what it means to be a nurse.

And of course, it's essential to offer opportunities. Internships, mentoring programmes, international exchanges; every experience is a window onto the vast world of nursing. These opportunities allow young aspiring nurses to see the many facets and specialisations of the profession, whether in neurosurgery, palliative care, oncology research or public health.

Finally, to inspire, you have to support. Nursing is a demanding profession, both physically and emotionally. It is therefore essential to put in place support structures, whether through discussion groups, continuing education or professional development opportunities.

Inspiring the next generation of dedicated nurses means painting a vivid picture of what it means to be a nurse today: a mix of science and humanity, challenge and reward, history and innovation. It's a call to all those with an open heart and a desire to make a positive difference in the world, one patient at a time.